Most Underappreciated

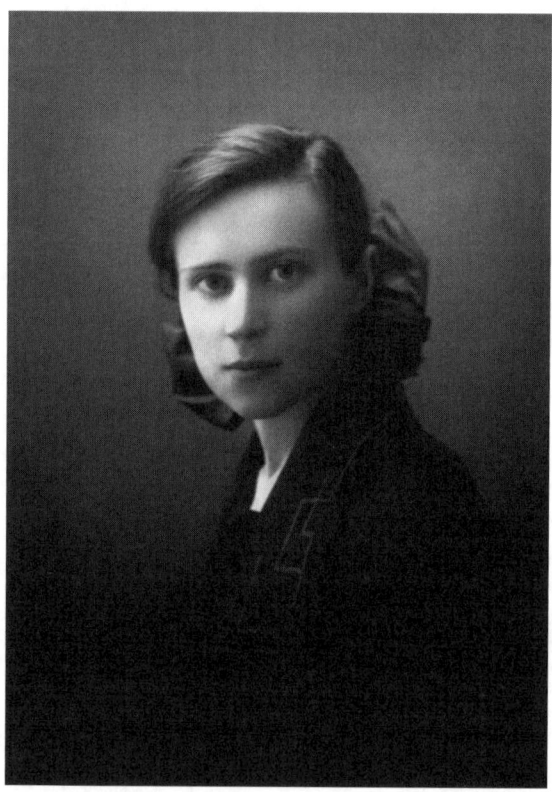

Bluma Zeigarnik, circa 1921. Born in 1901, Zeigarnik studied in the 1920s at the University of Berlin under the mentorship of Kurt Lewin (widely regarded as the father of modern social psychology) on essential aspects of his field theory, leading to her dissertation on what was later to become known as the "Zeigarnik Effect" (where she found that tasks interrupted are recalled approximately 90% better than those fully completed). In 1925, she graduated from university, and in 1927 was awarded the PhD. She returned to Moscow in 1931 and continued work as a neuropsychologist for 56 years, ultimately holding a chair in Neuropsychology at Moscow State University. Photo courtesy of her grandson Andrey Zeigarnik with permission of the Zeigarnik family.

MOST UNDERAPPRECIATED

*50 Prominent Social Psychologists
Describe Their Most Unloved Work*

Edited by Robert M. Arkin

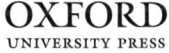
OXFORD
UNIVERSITY PRESS

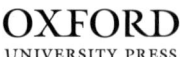

Oxford University Press, Inc., publishes works that further
Oxford University's objective of excellence in research,
scholarship, and education.

Oxford New York

Auckland   Cape Town   Dar es Salaam   Hong Kong   Karachi
Kuala Lumpur   Madrid   Melbourne   Mexico City   Nairobi
New Delhi   Shanghai   Taipei   Toronto

With offices in

Argentina   Austria   Brazil   Chile   Czech Republic   France   Greece
Guatemala   Hungary   Italy   Japan   Poland   Portugal   Singapore
South Korea   Switzerland   Thailand   Turkey   Ukraine   Vietnam

Copyright © 2011 by Oxford University Press, Inc.

Published by Oxford University Press, Inc.
198 Madison Avenue, New York, New York 10016

www.oup.com

Library of Congress Cataloging-in-Publication Data
Most underappreciated : 50 prominent social psychologists describe their most unloved work /
edited by Robert M. Arkin.
    p. cm.
  Includes bibliographical references.
  ISBN 978-0-19-977818-8 (pbk. : alk. paper) 1. Social psychology. I. Arkin, Robert M., 1950-
  HM1033.M67 2011
  302.092'2—dc22

                                                                    2010026118

Printed in the United States of America
on acid-free paper

To my teachers, friends, and cheerleaders: Jerry and Phil

PREFACE

Okay, so there are actually 55 essays, not 50, and 56 authors in all, as one essay is co-authored. Mea culpa, I suppose. I invited only a handful of others, early on, but those scholars either thought all their work was overappreciated, or they were just too busy to contribute something at the time. With 55 final invitations, I felt sure that a few people would have writer's block, get carpal tunnel syndrome, rethink their commitment, or miss a deadline. No one did.

The reason for this record-setting perfect attendance, I think, is that the idea for this book hit a chord with virtually everyone who stopped, even briefly, to think about the idea. This book is unique. Each essay is brief and to the point, and each essay serves a purpose—not merely for the reader, but for the author, as well.

For the author: This is a collection of reflections written by some of the most eminent social psychologists of this era. Each author was asked to describe some work she or he has published that just didn't hit the mark, didn't get the kind of attention it "should have," was misunderstood or misconstrued—what I described to them as their "most underappreciated" work. For some, it would be a matter of timing, publishing something before its time; for others a problem in the framing of the hypothesis or of the findings; for still others the publication outlet, the audience, and so forth. For some time, I have been asking visitors to Ohio State University informally, "What is your most underappreciated work?" and nearly without exception, people perk up and have a story to tell. As I asked this question, each conversation led to a dramatic change in my conversation partner's face, moving from a blank sort of "start," to a faint smile of recognition, a look into the middle distance, followed by a response that took a latency of only, perhaps, 10 seconds in all. Every such conversation (at least with senior scholars) led to a story, an illustration, a recounting of a project or idea—and a great story. As often as not, the story concerned a "monkey" that people had "on their backs." And so, this book offered the chance to right the ship of scholarship, to explain again more clearly, to correct a misapprehension, a misunderstanding, a mis-citation, and so forth. In short, writing a brief essay, for some, was an opportunity of a lifetime. The chance to get a monkey off one's back doesn't present itself every day.

My conversations with visitors often reminded me of the "Zeigarnik effect," which was first reported in the doctoral research of Bluma Zeigarnik (1927), a disciple of the Berlin Gestalt psychologists (Kohler, Wertheimer, and Lewin). She was an early PhD student of Kurt Lewin, who is generally regarded as the father of the discipline of social psychology. Zeigarnik found that people typically remember uncompleted tasks far better than completed tasks. Perhaps apocryphal, it has been said that the hypothesis emerged over a dinnertime conversation about servers in restaurants, who at the time were expected to recall patrons' orders at least until the bill was presented. My guess was that even these eminent psychologists had feelings of "unfinished business" about at least some of their work, and that I was hitting that "minor chord" with my invitation.

For the reader: I think the essays turned out to be even more delightful for the reader than they were unburdening for the authors. Some are "laugh out loud" funny and charming. Despite being written by some of the most eminent psychologists, one writer revealed that he has a published paper (in the flagship journal) that has *never* been cited—not even by himself! Another wrote that he has been trying to become a *social* psychologist for years and years, only to get the cold shoulder, even on the dance floor during after-meeting parties at conferences (that almost made me want to teach him the secret handshake). One writer mentioned a study inspired in part by The Who song "Pinball Wizard," and mentioned the dependent variable name "balls." One author, one of the nicest (and shortest) people you could ever meet, wrote about intellectual "sparring" and said she left meetings "bloodied, metaphorical sword still in hand … but jubilant that someone had engaged with the ideas."

Beyond the charm, the engaging stories, there is an intellectual objective as well, actually more than just one. The book is organized into five chapters:

- Big Science, Big Theory, Big Ideas
- Middle-Range Theories
- Methods and Innovations
- Phenomena and Findings
- Application: Making Science Useful

This organization means that the book covers the waterfront of social psychology. The essays span the same range of theories, methods, findings, and application as found in the typical social psychology textbook. The book is brief enough to be used as a supplement to a conventional textbook. And, for well-prepared students and those with some background, it could even serve as the core of a course. The theoretical, methodological, and practical matters raised make so many useful observations and touch on so much of the field that the book could serve profitably as the backbone of a "professional problems" course and be accompanied by readings.

To enhance the pedagogy, and to put a human face on the scholarly enterprise, each author was asked to address one of the four questions:

- Who were your mentors, or influential figures in psychology, that led you to study this particular question?

- What is important or useful about the theoretical framework that drove this research question?
- What advice would you offer for a new, young investigator, just entering the field, based on this work and your experience?
- What was the impact of this research on your own future research agenda?

This enabled people to write, with great affection, about their intellectual "North Stars" in a way that isn't usually available. There are fond recollections of Hal Kelley, Ned Jones, Don Campbell, Jud Mills, Jack Brehm, Michael Argyle, Jos Jaspers, Bob Zajonc, Fritz Heider, Stanley Schachter, and many more. And, of course, the Table of Contents reveals that the authors in this book are no less "North Stars" themselves; they are the luminaries of today. Many give advice to young scholars, the sort of guidance one could only get in casual conversation. The advice ranges from how to prepare for, and make the most of, a professorship in a liberal arts college context (where teaching is highly valued, perhaps more than research) to how to frame a research question, title an article, handle a controversy, pursue a passion, devise a method, think about a meta-analysis, write persuasively, and more.

Finally, and perhaps most engagingly, these eminent psychologists to a person made their professional lives a much more "human" and "social" enterprise than anyone usually knows or can see. Their stories are personal; they touch on relationships, people's passion about ideas, the emotional highs and lows of academic life, the parts of the "life of the mind" that get neglected in the sometimes dry, scientific prose that is the coin of the realm. These authors are all people who have enjoyed immense success. They are the sorts of scholars who typically do not let anything "go to press" unless they view it as a gem. But some of these expected gems are received in underwhelming ways, and it seems that even the leaders in our field don't quite get over that. This turns out to be a good thing, as their unfinished business (Zeigarnik, 1927) presents this chance to peer through the window and see how even the best and brightest are occasionally misunderstood, underappreciated, mis-cited, and, at least occasionally, missed entirely.

REFERENCE

Zeigarnik, B. (1927). Das Behalten erledigter und unerledigter Handlungen. *Psychologische Forschung, 9*, 1–85.

ACKNOWLEDGEMENTS

I thank my graduate school advisor and friend for more than three decades, Jerry Jellison, whose enthusiasm is contagious; his support is a continuous source of strength to me and his friendship through the years is an immeasurable gift. Both Jerry and Phil "Zim" Zimbardo, friend and teacher for two decades, were cheerleaders throughout this project, providing advice and an occasional push (sometimes followed by shove) to get it done.

I owe a huge debt of gratitude to Lori Handelman, Senior Editor at Oxford University Press, who saw the value in this project from the start. Her advice and counsel at every stage, start to finish, and her willingness to field incessant questions and lend her critical eye to all made her the best sounding board anyone could hope to have. Lori is not only a gifted thinker and writer generally, but her PhD in social psychology meant she knew all the "usual suspects" and she understands the field intimately, and I ultimately adopted the salutation Jedi Lori when writing her (as in "Dear JL").

Once this book was in production, Abby Gross took over where Lori left off and she was also a delight to work with; Ashley Polikoff was terrific in overseeing all of the project through production, and Joanna Ng and Anisha Shankar were both amazing in their detailed, professional work turning the manuscript in to a book. In every way, Oxford University Press proved a great organization populated by hardworking and really nice people! Thanks to all.

My oldest son, JD, and Uncle Bill, a Thanksgiving fixture in our home, listened first to my own story of being underappreciated, and didn't mind when I dashed off to get scratch paper and write out the idea for this book. The rest of the family didn't hear much from me during the busy times with deadlines, but they greeted incessant updates the rest of the time with good cheer, and even occasional interest.

The expectation that collecting these tales from colleagues would work stemmed, I think, from my many years of serving as a journal editor. I have routinely been amazed by the generosity and the thoughtful, clever, insightful things (yes, sometimes devastating) my colleagues have shared in their reviews of one another's work. This generous spirit of sharing what they know is what led me to believe such top-caliber scholars would contribute to this set of stories. So, I thank all those amazing scholars over the years for convincing me that social psychology is populated both by exceedingly bright and also very nice people who recognize that the whole to which they contribute is far greater than the mere sum of its parts.

Social psychologists are a talented, smart, sometimes smart-alecky, clever, and fun group of scholars who have remarkable insight into everyday life. I thank the authors of these essays, who rose to the occasion and who made these essays distinctly "human" and "social" and revealed something usually hidden in the scientific enterprise: a window onto how top-flight scholars think, act, and feel about their work.

Bob Arkin
Columbus, Ohio
June 2010

CONTENTS

Part V—Application: Making Science Useful   239

INTRODUCTION

MY OWN MOST UNDERAPPRECIATED RESEARCH

On Thanksgiving Day last year, Uncle Bill turned the conversation toward a topic at the natural intersection of the mind–body question that dogs philosophers and psychologists alike. He cited the statistics for air travel, that as many as 25% of flyers catch a cold from the shared, recirculated air in the plane. He then left the room briefly to get his Airborne, that relatively new product supposedly concocted by a teacher—those folks who are exposed to all manner of disease in their classrooms, and are therefore likely to be sick all the time. On his return he talked about his friends who insisted he use it to fend off a cold during all travel by air. My oldest son, on his first visit back home during his first quarter away at college (and consequently, knowing utterly everything, at least in his own mind), pointed to his head ... symbolizing that he guessed this was more about mind (that is, Uncle Bill's mind) than body. Really, I think he might have meant that Uncle Bill's mind was full of hot air.

Because my son, JD, was about to take Introductory Psychology his next quarter, and we rarely talk about my work or my spouse's work (she's a psychologist, too; poor kids) at home, I launched into a description of a set of studies that I noted was among my most underappreciated work.

Not that any of my work has changed the face of social psychology, or anything else, mind you, but I have had an eclectic set of interests over these 30 years, and I've done okay, even serving as a dean at Ohio State for 8 of those years, a journal editor for fully 14 of those years. The impact of my research has been variable, from getting some notice to receiving a little less.

Some of the least-noticed efforts are among the ones I am most proud of and pleased with, and this irony has been a source of amusement to me (and, I suppose, frustration) over the years. The idea for this book stems from that very moment and that conversation with my family and from my own nagging feeling that sometimes one's least appreciated work may be among what a scholar might see as his or her most "underappreciated" work. It isn't easy in the context of an article or chapter in a book always to say clearly why you think some idea, or set of data, is special, or huge, because there is not a lot of room to wax eloquent on that point. And, as they say, timing is everything. Sometimes one's work is out of time, or out of place. It may be before its time. It may be in a journal where the right set of scholars' eyes simply never see one's work, or it could be buried in a messy literature or read in the context of a literature that obscures the big "take-home point" that you see as most special.

I have had that experience more than once during my three-decades-long career. The one I described to my son that Thanksgiving Day was from the early 1980s. It was a "one-shot" effort that stemmed from long conversations between one of my most accomplished PhD students and me. Jerry Burger (now a professor at the Santa Clara University) was deeply invested in studying the psychology of control. He had published a scale on the Desire for Control with my friend and colleague Harris Cooper, and was working on a first book on the psychology of control. As time passed, literally dozens of articles on the topic came out of Jerry's lab at Santa Clara.

Our conversation was about learned helplessness. We talked at length about what would produce it, what might preclude it. Ultimately, the conversation landed on the question of what might inoculate people against succumbing to learned helplessness. Given our training, and the "Festinger tradition" that was our heritage, Jerry and I landed on a 2×2 conceptualization that independently explored the experience of predictability (present vs. absent) versus the experience of feelings of control (present vs. absent).

To that point, learned helplessness had been characterized as a response to loss of control, and the behavioral syndrome was (loosely) characterized as giving up, cowering, "throwing in the towel." Originally studied with animals, the absence of control would lead to passivity, cowering in the corner, and in people—to clinical depression.

Jerry and I noticed that, in all the research, the perception of predictability of events had been confounded with perceived control over those events. We explored the *independent* influence of perceived control and perceived predictability of an aversive event on participants' performance on a memory task, and their depressive affect that would result. Our guiding hypothesis was that, at least for people, predictability of aversive events might well be enough to provide inoculation against the nastiest effects of lack of control.

Participants received noise blasts that were both unpredictable and uncontrollable in one condition, and these individuals displayed performance deficits—and depressive affect about it—relative to a no-noise control group. However, participants who were able either to exert control over the noise blasts *or to have a measure of predictability* about the noise blasts did not show the same losses or depression. In short, either the sense of perceived control, or of perceived predictability, was sufficient to mitigate learned helplessness! Functionally, perceived control and perceived predictability were the same. Each inoculated our participants against the most maladaptive effects of learned helplessness.

In short, you don't necessarily have to enjoy complete control over events to avoid being a learned helpless basket case. For instance, when we go to the dentist, at least my dentist, I am always told something like "This is going to feel like a pinch, and might give you some discomfort" just before he injects a needle in my gums (a needle meant more for a Budweiser Clydesdale than for my gums, it seems to me). So, I clench my hands around the arm rests with my death grip. It's much the same when I am in a jetliner, taking off, and while I cannot control things any longer, I can at least grab my seat and tense up effectively. I am not fully learned helpless. I can prepare for aversive events. And while I don't have control, I enjoy the benefits of predictability.

We had a memorable exchange with Chuck Carver, who was then the editor of the personality section of the *Journal of Personality and Social Psychology*, the flagship journal for social psychology of the American Psychological Association. He really liked our distinction between predictability and control, and our idea that the two could be experimentally distinguished. He also liked our findings, and saw the results we uncovered as compelling support for distinguishing these two concepts and noting their independent impact, at least for humans.

However, the editor also had one (the one that we struggled the most with, and that I remember best) concern that nearly stumped us. He noted that it wasn't easy, and might not be possible, to think of a situation in daily life that reflected the presence of feelings of control (or the sensation of exerting control) but that was absent any sense of feelings of predictability. Chuck felt that publication of our work should probably depend at least in part on whether such a thing was possible (and, if not, then predictability and control were not truly orthogonal, or independent, in so-called real life).

Jerry and I talked endlessly about this, and eventually came up with our illustration. The editor was satisfied, the paper was published, and it... well... it seemed to land on deaf ears, despite being published in the flagship journal.

Our illustration was a person taking preventative or palliative cold medicine, which would convey a sense of exerting control over the viral infection known as the common cold. But taking the cold preventative/palliative at the outset of a cold doesn't convey anything about predictability. If you read on the label that something will cut the length of your cold in half, or cut your symptoms by a third, it is still entirely unclear what you can expect about the duration or debilitation of your cold. You get little in the way of predictability, and it's only the next morning when you wake that you can say with much confidence what you are likely to face for this particular cold—and then you're not certain.

I'm not sure about Jerry, but I thought this was one of the best insights linking "real life" with my work that I'd ever had. I had been taught that ecological validity was nice, but not a necessary precondition for doing quality thinking or excellent, important research. But there was something really energizing about solving this puzzle, and noting a pretty common experience of daily life that was a neat example of the conceptual distinction we made in the research.

Few readers saw its beauty. Not many cited our work. It was a "one-shot" study, which nearly everyone agrees is not the way to make you famous as a scholar, but gee… it was such an elegant study, and such a neat idea.

It was still a thrill to me to tell my son and Uncle Bill about the study, the idea, the totally fascinating original learned helplessness work of Seligman's that first stimulated our thinking. I had gotten my wife to tell about the original learned helplessness work, as her doctoral dissertation was on a cognitive aspect of the original work, extended to clinical psychology. It also gave me the opportunity to talk with my son about positive psychology, and Seligman's role in that, and then talk about my friends and colleagues and neighbors in our community here in Columbus, Ohio, and their influence, and how much my son was going to love psychology when he got started next quarter. In short, a side benefit of the 25 years of underappreciation that had stuck in my memory was an opening to talk with my son about the mind–body problem in general (he also took a beginning philosophy course that next quarter) and to connect with my son's educational experience and my own joy in learning. I'm sure it would be much nicer to have had the study Jerry and I published have a bigger impact, but this side benefit was not an all-bad substitute.

And during the conversation, I jotted down the idea for this book, so… things have a way of righting themselves, in the end.

Most Underappreciated

PART I

Big Science, Big Theory, Big Ideas

WALTER MISCHEL, Columbia University

Most Cited, Least Read?

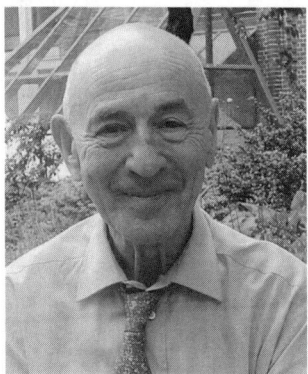

The greatest irony of my professional life is that my 1968 monograph *Personality and Assessment*, which brought me quick fame and even more infamy, is credited with causing an endless debate I found absurd from the start, splitting the two fields I hoped it would unite. It remains widely cited (more than 2500 citations), is still republished, and has been praised and hated for decades, generally for the wrong reasons, I suspect mostly by people who never read it, but keep discussing it in their textbooks and lectures, almost never quoting from it, not even paraphrasing. It would take a historian of science to figure out why it became the Rorschach card for so many colleagues on both sides of the social-personality hyphen, and still may serve that function, I hope less often. Perhaps my remarks here might encourage a few curious newcomers to psychological science to actually read it. But given its track record for 40 years, that's not likely—so at least take a look at the concluding paragraph from the book reputedly written to "kill personality" and undermine the role of individual differences:

> Global traits and states are excessively crude, gross units to encompass adequately the extraordinary complexity and subtlety of the discriminations that people constantly

make. . . . The traditional trait-state conceptualizations of personality, while often paying lip service to [people's] complexity and to the uniqueness of each person, in fact lead to a grossly oversimplified view that misses both the richness and the uniqueness of individual lives . . . [and their] extraordinary adaptiveness and capacities for discrimination, awareness, and self-regulation. (Mischel, 1968, p. 301)

Still strikes me as something that shouldn't have been too upsetting for personality psychology even 40 years ago, and I'd expect most everybody to quietly, even sleepily, nod and say "Sure, why not." Then why all the controversies with much sound and fury for so many years?

I first stumbled towards this book when I was a beginner teaching at Harvard in the Social Relations Department in 1960, preparing a survey course for graduate students in the personality program on the state of personality psychology and assessment. The deeper I got into the personality and assessment literature, most of which I had managed to avoid as a graduate student, the more I was surprised by the discrepancies between what the personality theories assumed and what the data showed. The theories assumed broad consistency in the individual's trait-relevant behaviors across diverse situations. But the gist of the data indicated that the aggressive child at home, for example, may turn out to be less aggressive than most when in school; the man exceptionally hostile when rejected in love may calmly accept criticism of his work; the one who dissolves anxiously in the dentist's office may be also be a courageous deep-sea diver; the bold risk-taking entrepreneur may shrink at his own cocktail parties. Research articles and doctoral dissertations often were reaching the same conclusions, but the disappointed investigators blamed themselves for the failure of their personality tests and their studies to yield the expected correlations. There was lots of "mea culpa" about poor methods and unreliable measures, but nobody questioned the key theoretical assumptions that guided them.

WHY THE TRAUMATIC FALLOUT FROM 1968?

The 1968 monograph traumatized many personality psychologists, I think, not because it called attention to the disappointing results of global trait-based personality assessment research that was already beginning to become clear. It was distressing because it asked: What if the problem is not just with bad methods and poor studies but also with wrong core assumptions? And I concluded that for a half-century researchers had been looking for personality guided by untenable assumptions, and therefore could not find the consistencies they expected. The fallout was that it left most personality psychologists with their paradigm down. Not a great way to make friends.

Upon publication the 1968 book was dismissed on a back page of *Contemporary Psychology*, in a short review titled "Personality Unvanquished," but within a year the "person versus the situation debate" exploded and dominated much of the agenda in personality and social psychology. This heated confrontation filled the journals' pages and the field's national and international meetings for more than 15 years, and deepened what to me was the absurd conceptual split between person and situation and between personality psychology and social psychology. Most personality psychologists reacted to the 1968 book as trivializing the importance of personality and overblowing the causal power of situations, and took it as a rejection of the "existence of personality" and the "power of the person." Most social psychologists cited it as proof for the "power of the situation" and the relative insignificance of individual differences in personality. In their debate, the two sides pitted the "power of the person" versus "the power of the situation," to argue about which was the bigger causal agent, which one accounted for more variance.

I thought both sides equally missed the point and the intended 1968 message. For years in subsequent papers I tried to make clear that I had always refused to ask "Is information about individuals more important than information about situations?" because phrased that way it is unanswerable and can only serve to stimulate futile polemics, in which "situations" are erroneously invoked as entities that supposedly exert either major or only minor control over behavior. The debaters kept on debating. The dispute took on its own life, further splitting social and personality psychology at exactly the most unnatural joints, severing the study of persons from the situations in which they functioned rather than focusing on their links and reciprocal interactions.

The result on one side was a "situationist" extremism that indeed trivialized the role of individual differences, and treated personality coherence as an illusion and an attribution error. On the other side, many personality psychologists renewed even more intensely their efforts to retain the traditional paradigm. They argued that global dispositions as traditionally conceptualized were "alive and well" if one simply aggregated multiple observations and measures across different situations. Thereby they again eliminated the role of the situation by averaging it out. This strategy now acknowledged that specific behaviors across different types of situations could not be predicted by such a model and simply continued to treat the situation as a source of noise by removing it as before.

As the debate escalated, so did the distance between what was said about the book that ostensibly caused it and the book's contents. In the 1980s I was not infrequently described by personality psychologists as the devil of the field who tried to destroy it, and "Mischel, 1968" was stuck into parentheses as the cited evidence. A multiple choice test item on a major state examination for many years was particularly upsetting to some of my students by asking them to identify the psychologist who "did not believe in personality," and making Mischel the right answer. It required short-term therapy from their mentor.

WHAT WAS IN THE 1968 BOOK? NOT *SAID* ABOUT IT, BUT *IN* IT?

Forty years after *Personality and Assessment* was published it was therefore a happy surprise to see that Orom and Cervone (2009) did something that almost never happens for the 1968 book: They did a scholarly review and systematic, quantitative content analysis of what's in it, not what gets said about it. Their analysis showed that the book consists of two halves: the first documents the challenges facing the field and some of the main limitations in the concepts and methods regnant at that time; the second:

> concerns psychological dynamics, cognitive processes, subjective meaning, and individual idiosyncrasy. In these pages, the book has little coverage of personality "traits" or "consistency"—topics commonly thought to have dominated Mischel's work. Our analysis indicates that . . . the point of his book was to advance a personality psychology that centered on psychological dynamics of meaning construction and that simultaneously was sensitive to the idiosyncrasies of the individual. (Orom & Cervone, 2009)

Orom and Cervone then underline that a key message of the 1968 book was that the assessor's focus needs to be on the particular meanings that stimuli and situations have acquired for the individual. They conclude their paper by making a point I have long hoped to see in the personality literature: "Whether you liked it or not, the first half of Mischel's famed volume did not argue that cross-situational consistency in personality functioning is low. It argued that cross-situational consistency in personality functioning is low when one searches for consistency through the lens of global, nomothetic trait constructs. When one tries on different lenses, things clear up" (Orom & Cervone, 2009).

FROM PARADIGM CHALLENGE TO PARADIGM ALTERNATIVE

Beginning in the late 1970s and early 1980s, the factor analytic approach was rediscovered to resuscitate the classic trait paradigm. It was reborn with an agreement (far from unanimous) among researchers about the major traits, dubbed the "Big Five," needed for a comprehensive taxonomy of personality, based on trait ratings. To me it looked like a 20-year regression supported by popular vote and acclamation, not by convincing new evidence, to return to business as usual. For many personality psychologists it soon became synonymous with the construct of personality itself. It was hard for me to believe that a model like the five-factor theory, a conception like the Big Five, and a measurement tool like the NEO-R, was really going to become equated with the very definition of personality. Was this field ready to have a view of the human being confined to such characterizations with trait adjectives that categorize people so simplistically? Was personality going to be split from the study of the self, of individual differences in how people think, feel, and process information about the social world? Was it going to be divorced from how what we think, feel, and do connects to what is around us, and links to how our brains work, even to how our genes play out? Put simply, I feared that the view of human personality in our science was in danger of becoming headless, brainless, self-less, de-contextualized from the social world, lacking an unconscious, and missing an emotional/motivational system.

THE MORAL OF THE STORY

The resurgence of the traditional trait approach in the form of the Big Five further spurred my desire, shared with Yuichi Shoda and many others, to go from challenging the paradigm to seeking a better alternative, and getting to the locus for the intuition that there surely is consistency or at least coherence in personality, but not where it had been assumed to be. Over many years, it was found by incorporating the situation into the assessment and conception of the individual, rather than by treating it as the error term. By including the situation as it is perceived by the person, and by analyzing behavior in this situational context, the consistencies that characterize the person, far from disappearing as had been assumed, began to be identified. We discovered that these individual differences are expressed not in consistent cross-situational behavior; instead, consistency is found in distinctive but stable patterns of *if ... then ...*, situation–behavior relations that form contextualized, psychologically meaningful cognitive-affective-behavioral signatures (e.g., "she does, thinks, feels A when X, but B when Y"). And these signatures of personality in turn begin to open windows into the underlying relatively stable processing system that generates them—the Cognitive Affective Processing System or CAPS that Yuichi Shoda and I outlined in our 1995 *Psychological Review* piece.

If there's a lesson to be learned from this story, perhaps it's that a paradigm challenge will either be ignored, or create a lot of noise and strife, but will change little until a better alternative emerges and gets a chance. Perhaps the 1968 challenge had some value, even for those who never read it, maybe by leading to a polarization that sharpened the issues, insisted they be confronted, and even pointed to the needed next steps. But to have a chance of changing anything, you need a paradigm alternative, lots of luck, great students and colleagues, dog-like persistence, and above all longevity. Yes, and tenure at a good university helps a lot. And then it takes another 40 years to see if any of it mattered or is remembered. But no matter how it plays out, it's still the best serious game in town.

REFERENCES

Mischel, W. (1968). *Personality and assessment*. New York: Wiley.
Orom, H., Cervone, D. (2009). Personality dynamics, meaning, and idiosyncrasy: Assessing personality architecture and coherence idiographically. [Special Issue] "Personality and Assessment 40 years later." *Journal of Research in Personality, 43*(2).

MARILYNN B. BREWER, University of New South Wales
Appreciated, but Misunderstood

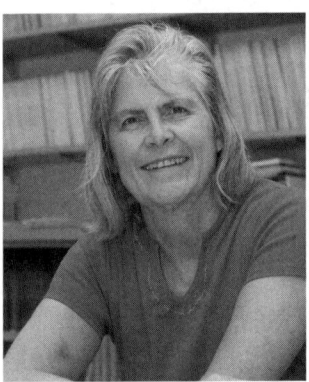

When I was first presented with the idea behind this volume, I thought it is probably true that most of us have felt that at least one of our pet ideas or research findings never received the attention or recognition that it deserved. But then I thought, why stop there? Aren't there also times when our good work languishes for far too long before it is finally noticed and acknowledged? Or, perhaps even more common, a paper is cited frequently but misquoted or misrepresented? I could think of examples of each of these forms of "underappreciation" and, with the encouragement of our stalwart editor, decided to make this chapter three-for-the-price-of-one.

MOST UNDERAPPRECIATED

My most underappreciated contribution was not a research finding but a concept that I tried to introduce to the field in a short commentary published in *American Psychologist* in 1976. The backdrop for the article was a longstanding debate between me (the upstart new PhD) and my brilliant mentor, Donald Campbell. Convinced by evolutionary biologists that humans, like other organisms, are genetically selfish,

Don believed that we had to look to the evolution of social institutions and power-ful cultural and religious traditions to understand the social achievements of human beings. These ideas culminated in the text of his presidential address to the American Psychological Association in 1975, where he argued that there is an inherent conflict between the forces of biological evolution (selecting for individual self-in-terest) and those of social evolution (providing external constraints on selfishness in the interests of group survival). It was on these points that Don and I had our most interesting and challenging disagreements. (Don encouraged such debates and urged his students to challenge his ideas, though he rarely actually changed his mind …) I just could not accept the idea that the extent of sociality and sustained group living that characterizes human beings could have been maintained solely by external constraints embodied in social institutions, traditions, and practices selected at the group level and operating in opposition to biological selection.

I expressed my disagreement in print in a short comment on his presidential address (Brewer, 1976) where I argued that the profound ambivalence between personal self-gratification and self-sacrifice for collective welfare is not a conflict between internal biological motives and external social constraints but rather an internal biological dualism that reflects human evolutionary history as a social spe-cies. My point was that human beings are neither inherently purely selfish nor purely altruistic but instead are characterized by a kind of functional antagonism between self-interested and group-interested behavior. Because of the resultant variability in motives underlying human social behavior, I suggested, the distribu-tion of human sociality might best be depicted in terms of a "golden standard devia-tion" rather than a "golden mean."

Personally, I thought that the "golden standard deviation" was an elegant idea that would surely be picked up widely and would revolutionize social psychologists' approach to the study of social motivation. But, alas, its brilliance was never recog-nized and no revolution took place on the heels of my little commentary. (I did, however, resurrect the construct several years later in the form of optimal distinc-tiveness theory [Brewer, 1991], which did get its share of recognition.)

MOST DELAYED APPRECIATION

Another legacy of Don Campbell's mentorship was my involvement in the Cross-Cul-tural Study of Ethnocentrism project, which was ongoing during my graduate student days at Northwestern University. The CCSE was a unique, ambitious interdisciplinary project that combined ethnographic data collection in remote stateless societies around the world and survey data collection among 30 tribes in East Africa. The East African data became the basis for my dissertation research project and culminated in the publication of a book summarizing our findings on ethnocentric attitudes and intergroup perception in post-colonial East Africa (Brewer & Campbell, 1976). The uniqueness of the data, its historical context, and its relevance for the social psychology of intergroup relations should have garnered a reasonable amount of attention in the field, but, again, the book went out of print after a few short years, with a couple of citations by cross-cultural psychologists but barely a notice in the social psychology literature (apparently 1976 was a bad year for me …).

You can imagine my surprise, then, when more than 15 years later citations to *Ethnocentrism and Intergroup Attitudes: East African Evidence* began showing up in my annual Social Science Citation Index (SSCI) record. How it happened that a long-out-of-print book was resurrected from the moribund provides an interesting case study in the sociology of science.

One factor was the historical context that shapes and channels research interests in a field like social psychology. During the Cold War era and following the major civil rights movement activities of the 1950s and 60s, various forms of regional, religious, and ethnic intergroup conflict were either ignored or believed to be largely resolved, and social psychologists lost interest in the study of intergroup relations as a mainstream endeavor. Social cognition was on the rise and, like almost everyone else in the field, I retreated to the laboratory to study person memory and reaction times to process social information. By 1990, however, the complacency about the state of intergroup relations in the world had been shattered. The demise of the Soviet Union and the apparent resurgence of ethnic conflicts throughout the world gave rise to the idea that local group loyalties and intergroup hostilities were never far below the surface. The media began talking about the "new tribalism" that seemed to be emerging everywhere. As public interest in these issues grew, so did a resurgence of interest in theory and research on intergroup relations within social psychology, in Europe and in the U.S. In that context, the study of intergroup attitudes and ethnocentric bias was suddenly a hot topic again.

The second factor was technological—the introduction of search engines and massive online bibliographic databases. With little effort, a social psychologist with a new-found interest in ethnocentrism and ingroup bias could type those terms into his or her online search and out would pop Brewer and Campbell (1976). I have no idea how many people actually read the book, but the citations are gratifying, even if overdue.

APPRECIATED BUT MISUNDERSTOOD

According to SSCI, my 1988 lead article in *Advances in Social Cognition* ("A dual process model of impression formation") has been cited more than 500 times (by authors other than me) in the two decades since its publication. And my estimate is that well more than half of those citations got it just plain wrong. The paper is frequently cited in connection with the idea that social category stereotypes dominate person perception and impression formation and that stereotyping is the low-effort default process for encoding and remembering social information. Ironically, the article was written to counter that very idea by positing instead that there are two distinct modes of processing social information—a category-based (top-down) processing mode and a person-based (bottom-up) processing mode. In order to be especially provocative, I postulated that the two modes of processing not only differed in the way information was attended to and encoded but also resulted in different forms of mental representation. Neither processing mode was presumed to be primary, but each depended instead on the perceiver's goals, intentions, and relationship to the target person. Even when the target person is identifiable as a member of a salient social category, the dual process model assumes that category stereotypes will not be accessed or utilized when a strong interpersonal orientation characterizes the relationship between perceiver and target.

A related misconception of the dual process model is to equate category-based and person-based processing with heuristic versus systematic, elaborative processing, respectively. As opposed to a single-mode sequential model of depth of processing of social information, my dual process model assumed that perceivers can use heuristic or elaborative processing in either mode. When effortful processing is engaged, both category-based and person-based modes result in individualized impressions of the target person, but the dual process model distinguishes between individuated impressions that are the product of category-based processing and personalized impressions that result from bottom-up person-based processing.

Although it is disappointing that many citers of Brewer (1988) miss the central point of the theory, to be honest, I have to take responsibility for making the point less clear than it should have been. The paper as a whole is densely written, with multiple paths for the reader to try to follow. And I made the mistake in one section of the paper of referring to different components of the model as "stages," which paved the way for misrepresentation as a single sequential model. (From this point forward, I encourage future readers or re-readers of the article to focus on Figure 1.1 and ignore Table 1.1.) In any case, the consequence has been that although Brewer (1988) has received its share of citations, the primary intended idea of the paper remains among the "most unappreciated."

REFERENCES

Brewer, M. B. (1976). Comment on Campbell's "On the conflicts between biological and social evolution." *American Psychologist, 31*, 372.

Brewer, M. B. (1988). A dual process model of impression formation. In T. Srull & R. Wyer (Eds.), *Advances in Social Cognition* (Vol. 1, pp. 1–36). Hillsdale, NJ: Erlbaum.

Brewer, M. B. (1991). The social self: On being the same and different at the same time. *Personality and Social Psychology Bulletin, 17*, 475–482.

Brewer, M. B., & Campbell, D. T. (1976). *Ethnocentrism and intergroup attitudes: East African evidence.* New York: Halsted Press (Sage Publications).

MAHZARIN R. BANAJI, Harvard University
Undeserved Recognition

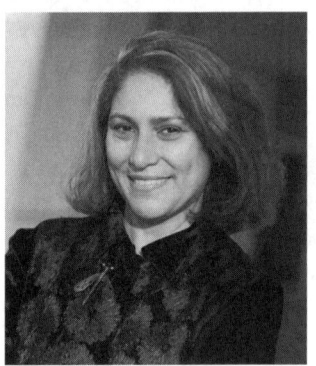

*B*ill McGuire, my colleague at Yale for 15 years, would mail his reprints in response to requests with some version of this message scrawled on letterhead: "For those of you whose lips move when you read JPSP, consider wearing sun glasses when you read this to shield yourself from the glare of the brilliance of these words." It was never fully clear whether he was poking fun at himself while skewering a novice (like me), or whether he was subtly signaling that his work had not received the recognition it deserved.

Since 1980, the year I started graduate school, I have sat in an intellectual rotunda filled with remarkable colleagues in every direction. Nobody could question that they each had received enormous recognition, and in many cases, complete adoration as well. But even gods feel underappreciated, I learned, and being a keen observer of them, I have, for the past three decades, waited for the moment when I too would get in a huff and dash off a note about the dull pupillary reflexes of some poor reader. But alas, that occasion hasn't presented itself. I do not deserve to be in this book. Moreover, the reception to my work has corresponded pretty well to my own sense of it. The work I've regarded to be relatively more shiny has also been more recognized than the work I myself have regarded to be less radiant. Not only has nothing been forgotten or unappreciated, there has been a sufficiently reassuring correspondence in self–other perception of the work. So, as I said, I don't deserve to be in this book.

In fact, the contrary has been true. Some papers that I thought would have gathered dust have actually received more attention than they have deserved. On one occasion, a long time ago, I wrote a paper with my colleague Robert Crowder stating that the "practical aspects of memory" movement had made the mistake of equating the use to which basic research is put with research that employs seemingly realistic methods (Banaji & Crowder, 1989). Maybe it was the tone of the paper that created a ruckus; it started this way:

> Once upon a time, when chemistry was young, questions of ecological validity were earnestly raised by well-respected chemists, and were debated at scientific meetings and in scholarly journals. We understand from a colleague (who is a distinguished historian of science but modestly asked not to be named) that partisans of one point of view called themselves the "Everyday Chemistry Movement." They pointed out that the world offered many vivid examples of chemical principles at work in our daily lives—the rising of pastry dough, the curdling of sauces (the great chef Brillat-Savarin was then laying the foundation for the principles of applied chemistry called thereafter French cuisine), the smelting of metal alloys, the rusting of armor, and the combustion of gunpowder. Why not, they asked, study chemical principles in these ecologically faithful settings rather than in tiresome laboratories with their unnatural test tubes, burners, and finicky rules of measurement? The normal world around us, they said, has no end of interesting and virtually unstudied manifestations of chemistry. (p. 1185)

Tongue in cheek, we narrated the obvious oddity of arguing that a science should strive to make itself look ecologically valid to naïve observers. Surely no biologist would argue that we should set aside the use of *C. elegans*, a worm that lives for 2 to 3 weeks, as the preparation to understand development, genetics, aging, and disease because *C. elegans* doesn't look much like us. In this paper on the study of memory we said nothing terribly profound; just the sort of thing one would say to coach a high school debate team preparing to make a case about the value of the scientific method and the role of basic research in solving practical problems. What nonsense all this practical methods stuff was in the context of understanding human memory, we said, and ended with a harrumph. And then we went to bed like any other day. When we awoke, a tea-party–like mob had formed on both sides of the Atlantic and an issue of *American Psychologist* had been devoted to responses to that paper, mainly critical, with one exception by Roddy Roediger, who stuck his neck out for us. I had only completed my second year as assistant professor at the time, but I had to duck with the swiftness of President Bush dodging a shoe at the next Psychonomics meeting I attended. Fame was one thing, but not at the expense of taking a few stitches in the head.

Many years later, another colleague at Yale described my apparently perceptive use of the early years to write theoretical rather than empirical papers because Yale's subject pool was so small I couldn't do much research. I'm pretty sure that no such advance planning went into the decision to write that paper. It just seemed like the right thing to do, not to mention fun, but I had no idea it would get the undeserved attention it did. It brought me many reprint requests, most of them from the many amazing teachers of psychology at non-research institutions who told me horror stories of the difficulty of getting people to understand the value of basic research. And it brought from those who felt attacked a strong and personal sense of being harmed that I did not understand. (One very famous psychologist who I admired greatly told me he would not shake my hand at that Psychonomics!)

I learned a lot from the response to that paper. I learned that although I had no stomach for interpersonal conflict, I was unflappable when disagreements concerned intellectual matters, no matter how severe. The experience of writing that paper gave me the opportunity to spar. I would leave meetings bloodied, metaphorical sword still in hand, but jubilant that somebody had engaged with the ideas. I also learned that people didn't expect tough words to emerge from the body of a smallish, brown-skinned woman who seemed reasonably nice when you met her. A gender stereotype was being disconfirmed in a small way, and how could I not be in heaven over that too.

Another occasion on which I experienced undeserved attention wasn't in the context of a single paper but rather in the response to a body of work on implicit social cognition. My colleagues and I said what everybody else before us had already said: *Thinking and feeling can operate without conscious awareness. Therefore, mental states have consequences that are not intended. You, not just those "other" subjects in some textbook psychology experiment, may be prone to this.* That's it. Perhaps because we used black Americans and not green peas as attitude objects, the shoes came flying again. We were asked what hubris had led us to make a website and invite anybody and everybody to sample what we had learned about our own unconscious biases in the areas of social group attitudes. By now, I had rheumatoid arthritis and couldn't duck as fast as President Bush when the shoes came flying. But again, the experience was nothing short of exhilarating. Some pretty remarkable people put aside the primary work of their own careers to devote time to challenging our point of view. What more can one ask? I had certainly not done the same for them. I seem to have gained enormously, yet again, from this undeserved recognition.

REFERENCE

Banaji, M. R., & Crowder, R. G. (1989). The bankruptcy of everyday memory. *American Psychologist, 44*, 1185–1193.

ELLEN BERSCHEID, University of Minnesota

Is There a Divorce in Your Genes?

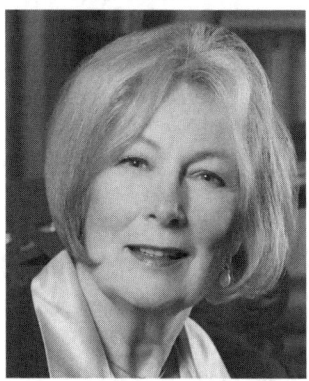

Using the classical twin method, the methodological mainstay of investigations of the relative contributions of genetic and environmental influences on human behavior, McGue and Lykken (1992) concluded that divorce is heritable: "The robustness and magnitude of the MZ-DZ [monozygotic–dizygotic twins] difference in divorce concordance indicates a strong influence of genetic factors in the etiology of divorce" (p. 368). They speculated that heritable personality characteristics associated with divorce mediate the association.

The assertion that divorce is heritable was of interest to many social psychologists, for we have been interested in the stability of interpersonal relationships, especially marital and other romantic relationships, for a very long time. When the authors asked me to comment on a pre-publication draft of their manuscript, I responded that a causal condition known to influence the stability of romantic relationships is the quality of alternatives to the relationship that exist in the individual's social environment (e.g., one study found that a spouse's perception of the goodness of his or her alternatives to the marital relationship predicted divorce significantly better than the individual's satisfaction with the marriage [Udry, 1981]). In addition, I continued, social psychologists also had amply demonstrated that an individual's goodness of alternatives to his or her romantic relationship is influenced by that individual's level of physical attractiveness; physically attractive people have more and better romantic relationship alternatives than the unattractive do. Thus, if MZ ("identical") co-twins are more similar in physical attractiveness than DZ ("fraternal") co-twins, then divorce concordance could be the result of an interaction between a heritable morphological variable, physical attractiveness, and a social environmental variable—namely, a society that values physical attractiveness. If so, divorce would not be found to be heritable by their method in a society in which physical attractiveness was not highly valued. I expressed concern that if their manuscript was published without caveat, some consumers of their report would worry that their genes doomed them to divorce, while others would happily absolve themselves of personal responsibility for dissolving their marriages in a "I can't help it—the genes made me do it" fashion. In fact, I promised them a steak dinner if the media did not publicize their study with a "divorce is in the genes" headline. I did not have to buy the dinner. On the heels of publication of their study, *USA Today* published an account of it under the headline "Half of All Divorces May Be Due to Genes."

The validity of the twin method for estimating the heritability of a behavior rests on the Equal Environments Assumption (EEA), which assumes that MZ and DZ co-twins are exposed to the same environmental influences and, thus, greater behavioral similarity among MZ co-twins relative to DZ co-twins is caused by the MZ co-twins' greater genetic similarity. If MZ co-twins' environments are more similar than those of DZ co-twins, the EEA is violated and heritability estimates are compromised.

Much of the controversy surrounding the twin method has focused on the validity of the EEA. Most twin method proponents now acknowledge that the environments of MZ co-twins may be more similar than those of DZ co-twins in several respects but argue that the twin method may be used if it can be shown that the environmental features that show a difference are *not causally associated* with the behavior of interest. Adherents of this modification of the EEA, termed the "equal trait-relevant environments assumption" (ETREA), argue that it has not been established that associations exist between the several known differences in the similarity of MZ and DZ twin pairs' environments and the behaviors they have investigated. Nevertheless, some behavior geneticists have recognized the potential threat of differences between MZ and DZ co-twins in similarity of physical attractiveness and have conducted a few studies that have led to acceptance of the null hypothesis of "no difference" in physical attractiveness similarity of MZ and DZ co-twins and have declared the EEA intact on this count.

My student, Matt Heller, and I noted that the few investigations of differences in similarity of attractiveness between MZ and DZ co-twins had very low statistical power to detect a difference. As every psychology student knows, small samples, scales of unknown or dubious reliability, and weak statistics make it easy for anyone who wishes to confirm the null hypothesis to do so, which is why such confirmations usually are of little value. On the other hand, we reasoned, perhaps it is true that no such difference exists. Although MZ co-twins are obviously more similar in physical appearance than DZ co-twins, the latter could well be more dissimilar in appearance but not dissimilar in physical attractiveness, for two facially dissimilar people can both be unattractive or attractive (e.g., think George Clooney and Brad Pitt).

Heller and I believed the question deserved an adequate test, for if MZ co-twins are significantly more similar in physical attractiveness than DZ twins, then the "goodness of alternatives" feature of their social environments, known to be causally related to relationship stability, would be significantly different, and the ETREA would be violated for calculating heritability estimates of divorce and, also, for the other social behaviors known to be associated with physical attractiveness. If a test of sufficient power to detect a difference did not find one, this controversial issue would be settled.

Matt McGue graciously agreed to allow us access to Minnesota Twin Registry photos under conditions of extreme confidentiality in order that we might investigate the degree to which MZ, DZ, and ZZ (zero zygosity) pairs shared facial similarity and facial physical attractiveness level using a sufficiently large twin sample, which, along with a sufficient number of raters, a highly controlled judgment setting, and reliable scales, provided ample statistical power to detect differences if they existed. The physical attractiveness of each twin was evaluated independently of the physical attractiveness level of his or her co-twin using a procedure designed to keep raters of the photos blind to the fact that they were assessing twins (see Heller & Berscheid, 2006).

Overall, the twins in the MZ sample did not differ in physical attractiveness level from the twins in the DZ sample but, as we suspected, the physical attractiveness levels of MZ co-twins were significantly more similar than those of DZ co-twins. We concluded that the social environments of MZ co-twins are likely to be more similar than those of DZ co-twins on the basis of their greater similarity in facial attractiveness alone (the difference likely would have been even larger if their similarity on other morphological dimensions, such as height and physique, could have been taken into consideration). As a consequence, we argued, the validity of the ETREA is challenged for heritability estimates of those social behaviors known to be influenced by an individual's physical attractiveness level. We also noted that heritability estimates derived from studies of twins raised apart (adoption studies) do not escape violations of the ETREA arising from differential similarity of MZ and DZ co-twins' social environments on the basis of their differential degree of physical attractiveness similarity, because whether geographically close or distant, individuals of similar attractiveness levels are likely to experience, from the cradle to the grave, social environments that are more similar with respect to preferential treatment by others.

Although we expected both social psychologists and behavior geneticists to welcome definitive evidence on a point subject to much speculation and controversy, our study was so "underappreciated" it never saw the light of day. The reasons given added insult to the injury of rejection by social psychology's premier journal. The first objection cited in the editor's rejection letter revealed that it was not just our study that was being rejected but social psychology itself, to wit: "Reviewer 1 questions whether there really is conclusive evidence that 'differences in physical attractiveness level cause differences in social environments' and that 'differences in social environments cause differences in social behaviors and outcomes.'" Say what? Social psychology is commonly defined as the "study of social influence on behavior" and we social psychologists have delineated myriad ways in which "differences in social environments cause differences in social behaviors and outcomes." But, of course, and as one (non-social) psychologist who read our reviews observed, one does not have to be familiar with the social psychological literature to know "there is a reason that Chinese children speak Chinese and not English!"

Other cited objections to our study were almost as disconcerting. For example, the editor's summary letter stated: "The fact that MZ twins are more similar in terms of physical attractiveness than DZ twins comes across as "almost a tautology" in the words of Reviewer 1, or, in the words of Reviewer 3, seems true by definition." Really? Is this why behavior geneticists been so eager to declare that the difference doesn't exist? Or, if these reviewers assume the difference *does* exist by definition, how is it that the validity of the EEA is not compromised? Oh right!.... we forgot the first objection—namely, that even if the attractiveness similarity difference exists it doesn't matter because "there isn't conclusive evidence that differences in social environments cause differences in social behaviors and outcomes."

Disappointed, we took a lesson from the film *Meatballs* in which Bill Murray revived the spirits of his team of dejected losers by leading them in the chant "It just doesn't matter! It just doesn't matter! It just doesn't matter!" We, too, concluded that perhaps it just doesn't matter that our paper was rejected. Since we began our study, which took years to conduct, the usefulness of the classical twin method has become widely questioned, if not altogether discredited. For example, shortly after the rejection of our manuscript, the method received a withering critique in *Dædalus*, the Journal of the American Academy of Arts and Sciences; Ehrlich and Feldman (2007) noted, as others have, that many assumptions about twins inflate twin-based estimates of broad-sense heritability. One of these inflationary assumptions, they observe, is the EEA. As an example, they state that "factors in the nonfamilial environment of identical twins are often more similar than those of fraternal twins but this difference between identical and fraternal twins is usually ignored" (p. 7). In another context, but pertinent to our study, they comment: "Further it is well known that physical attributes of people greatly influence how other people treat them. Individuals with identical genomes are usually strikingly alike in appearance, and within the same culture they will be treated more similarly than randomly selected individuals of the same gender from the same occupational and age groups" (p. 8). "Well known" to some but not all, we discovered.

More importantly, Ehrlich and Feldman observe that "We now know more than enough about the human genome and human development to see that the notion of 'genes for behaviors' is misguided. . . . It is clear that when genes influence traits, including behaviors, they only do so in ways that are affected by environments." They conclude their critique by stating that "the claim that genes program our behaviors or, indeed, that genes are responsible for some specified fraction of any human behavior" is "ridiculous" (p. 12).

If any investigator wishes documentation that MZ and DZ co-twins do differ significantly in similarity of physical attractiveness level, the Heller and Berscheid (2006) manuscript, along with the editor's rejection letter, is available from the junior author. If any investigator (or reviewer for a social psychology journal) needs documentation that social environments influence human behavior, a social psychology textbook should be purchased. Among the mountains of evidence that social environments do influence human behavior will be citations to book-length compendiums and meta-analytic studies of the thousands of studies that detail how the social environments of the physically attractive differ from the social worlds of those of lesser attractiveness and how those environmental differences influence their behavior and their lives.

REFERENCES

Ehrlich, P., & Feldman, M. W. (2007). Genes, environments & behaviors. *Dædalus*, 136 (Spring), 5–12.

Heller, M. A., & Berscheid, E. (2006). *Heritability estimates of social behaviors: The physical similarity threat to the Equal Environment Assumption.* Unpublished manuscript, University of Minnesota.

McGue, M., & Lykken, D. T. (1992). Genetic influence on risk of divorce. *Psychological Science, 3,* 368–373.

Udry, J. (1981). Marital alternatives and marital disruption. *Journal of Marriage and the Family, 43,* 889–897.

TODD F. HEATHERTON, Dartmouth College

A Life-Changing Paper? That Depends on Your Interpretation

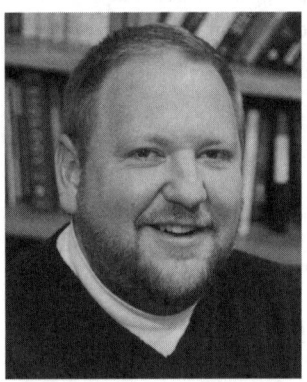

When asked to identify my most underappreciated paper, I pretty much knew right away which one I would write about. But that did not stop me from spending hours examining the *Web of Science* to see which of my papers were truly ignored—I found one from my early days that has never been cited, not even by me, not even by my three co-authors, not even a single time. My temptation to cite it here is trumped by the necessity of limiting citations to three; it will therefore remain in oblivion. Instead, the paper that I've often thought was underappreciated examined how people create and maintain life change by constructing narratives about how and why they changed (Heatherton & Nichols, 1994). In fairness, the paper has been cited about three times per year on average (total citations = 46), so it has not been totally ignored (although at least one recent paper in *JPSP* on narrative life change failed to cite it, so at least those authors support my claim of underappreciation). Here I describe why I wrote the paper, what we found, the story that we should have emphasized, and why I think we have a lot more to learn about how subjective interpretations are crucial for understanding life change.

NARRATIVE ACCOUNTS OF SUCCESSFUL AND UNSUCCESSFUL LIFE CHANGE

Whether people can change key aspects of their lives is a fascinating and important question for psychologists and the lay public alike. A glance at the psychology section in most bookstores (perhaps more appropriately called the *self-help* section) suggests that many people are trying to transform central aspects of their lives, such as getting over shyness, losing weight, giving up addictions, learning to like themselves, and so forth. Indeed, the life change industry is big business, raking in billions a year: self-help books bring in more than $10 billion, weight loss programs more than $50 billion, alcoholism treatment around $22 billion, and so on. The human species has amazing talents that have led to the development of higher education, space travel, medical miracles, and eye-popping technologies. But as my colleagues and I have noted over the years, people are also prone to self-regulatory failures, from failing at weight loss, to overcoming addictions, to avoiding driving while impaired, to spending beyond their means, etc. Thus, the life change industry benefits from a lot of repeat customers.

Given its importance, one might expect that understanding the psychological basis of life change would be a high priority for research. Yet this has not been the case, perhaps because studying life change is extraordinarily difficult. For instance, typically the evidence for change is obtained after it has taken place—even in prospective studies where there are assessments at various time points (and objective indicators might verify that change has occurred), there remains ambiguity regarding most aspects of change, such as time course (slow vs. sudden), differential motives, precipitating or sustaining factors, cognitive change, and so on. Indeed, although there are various theories about how people contemplate change, the factors that increase the likelihood of success (e.g., social support, an empirically validated psychological treatment, financial resources), and the conditions under which change is maintained, there is a stark lack of information regarding how people actually transform their thoughts, emotions, and behaviors. At the same time, in spite of the difficulties of understanding change, a variety of evidence indicates that people do make important life changes, both with and without therapy. But how do they do it?

To understand the phenomenology of life change, my graduate student Patricia Nichols and I collected narrative accounts from people who had succeeded at making major life changes versus accounts from people who had tried and failed in their attempts (Heatherton & Nichols, 1994). Because the paper is lightly cited and probably not widely read (hence its status as underappreciated), I will describe the basic findings. The successful and unsuccessful change stories differed in substantial and predictable ways. Individuals who reported successfully making changes described extreme negative affect, and often suffering, before the change was made, after which they developed a new identity. One common theme in the successful change stories was the occurrence of a focal event that triggered the change attempt, such as one woman deciding to leave her husband after taking a class that she said changed her entire outlook on life. Of course, we had no evidence that the change stories were true, and we speculated that people were misremembering their prior circumstances in order to create the perception that they had changed. We proposed that the stories people create may serve as important guides for future behavior. That is, the belief that one has changed may motivate behaviors that help sustain change.

UNCONSCIOUS FORCES AND THE INTERPRETER

One of the most important developments in psychology over the past few decades has been the growing recognition that much of human mental life exists below conscious awareness and that people are generally unaware of the cognitive processes (and the neural activity that gives rise to thought and emotion) that underlie most actions. Classic work by Richard Nisbett and Timothy Wilson demonstrated that people have limited access to their mental processes. Building on that seminal work, psychologists (notably John Bargh, Dan Wegner, and Ap Dijksterhuis) have documented important ways in which subtle, unconscious influences have a huge impact on behavior. Thus, contextual cues may prime certain thoughts or behaviors, such as viewing other people as more likeable when we are drinking a hot beverage. In Dan Wegner's elegant work, he has demonstrated that people have illusions of agency in which they either falsely believe they have control over events that occur without their involvement or lack a feeling of will for events they clearly did cause. This is important because it shows there can be a discrepancy between the actual cause of events and what people believe about the cause of those events. Hence, we begin with the idea that a great deal of behavior occurs in the absence of self-awareness of the mental processes underlying the behavior as well as possible misperceptions of personal agency for producing the behavior.

As has long been noted by attribution theorists, even with a lack of insight and inaccurate perceptions of agency, the human mind seems compelled to offer some explanation for events. The history of psychology has documented that people seem motivated to do two things: (1) make sense of events in a way that creates order and structure to instill a sense of coherency and predictability, and (2) portray the self in the best possible light. It is with these two motives in mind that we begin to understand the role of people's interpretations of events in relation to their perceived success or failure at life change. Let's examine the two motivational processes.

In terms of making sense of ongoing events, I have been greatly influenced by my collaborator Michael Gazzaniga's interpreter theory, based on his groundbreaking work with split-brain patients, whose two hemispheres had been surgically separated. In such patients, the left and right hemispheres can be interrogated separately by presenting information selectively to one or the other. Because there is contralateral control of movement (i.e., the right hemisphere controls the left side of the body and vice versa), the left hand can select an object that was shown to the right hemisphere, but the right hand cannot because it does not know what the right hemisphere observed. Mike identified a left hemisphere interpretive mechanism that creates causal explanations for events and actions, even in the absence of complete or veridical knowledge. For instance, in one classic study in which a split-brain patient's left hemisphere was forced to make sense of why the left hand selected a shovel (which was selected because it matched a snow scene shown to the right hemisphere), the left hemisphere (which was shown only a chicken claw) was quick to explain the action by the information available only to it, which is that the shovel must be used to clean out a chicken shed. In other words, when faced with personal actions for which the self does not have access to the mental and biological processes that produced them, the interpreter spins a story to make sense of events. Unfortunately, the interpreter's story is only as good as the material it has to work with, and as noted earlier, people have only limited access to the mental events that cause actions.

In terms of the motives to cast the self in a positive light, research in social psychology demonstrates that people's accounts of past events strongly influence their current self-perceptions as well as their assessments of whether they have changed. Anne Wilson and Michael Ross have conducted elegant research documenting the ways in which people disparage their past selves in order to bolster or enhance their current self-views (Ross & Wilson, 2003). This work builds on Michael Ross's earlier work showing that people get what they want by revising what they had (e.g., when you don't lose weight you might believe you did because you mistakenly recall that you used to be heavier than you are now). In other words, people distort their pasts to feel better with their present states. Likewise, Lisa Libby and her colleagues demonstrated that people think they have changed more when they consider themselves from the third-person perspective compared to the first-person perspective (Libby, Eibach, & Gilovoch, 2005). Libby and colleagues point out that subjectivism influences how people interpret change, a finding that is very consistent with that of our underappreciated paper.

PULLING IT TOGETHER

The various perspectives highlighted in this chapter (unconscious influence, left hemisphere interpreter, motivated reflections of the past) are key ingredients to understanding how people understand and describe their efforts at life change. As we speculated, it seems likely that a variety of forces conspire to produce change, only some of which are apparent to the person undergoing change. As the subjective interpreter examines the available evidence to make sense of things, and given the self-enhancement biases inherent in retrospective accounts, a story emerges that explains the life change in a way that portrays the past self as horribly flawed and the new self as changed in identity and distant from that flawed self.

Importantly, whether this interpretive account is accurate may not be important for future behavior. Put another way, irrespective of the factors actually responsible for change, what sustains change is dependent on the interpretive account. As William Thomas said in 1928, "If men define situations as real, they are real in their consequences." The belief that one has made a successful life change emerges from a narrative that explains the new self as changed in meaningful ways from one's old self. The implications of this pattern are important for understanding any endeavor in which people try to change. For instance, insight therapies may be unsuccessful because trying to get in touch with your real self and the past that produced that self may inadvertently affirm the core self that is difficult to change. Therapies such as cognitive behavior therapy might inspire the person to change to the person he or she wants to be and to break clear from the maladaptive past. Likewise, encouraging people to distance themselves from their old selves, in part by taking a third-person perspective, may help provide the resources to sustain the new self (Libby et al., 2005).

So, why was the original paper overlooked or underappreciated? I think the paper was a bit ahead of its time and did not benefit from the newer insights into unconscious processes, illusions of agency, constructive processes, and interpretive motives. Moreover, crossing levels of analysis from social to neurological accounts helps complete the story in a more satisfying way.

Then again, maybe my old self was a crappy writer with a bad sense of where to publish. Thank goodness I've changed.

REFERENCES

Heatherton, T. F., & Nichols, P. A. (1994). Personal accounts of successful versus failed attempts at life change. *Personality and Social Psychology Bulletin, 20,* 664–675.

Libby, L. K., Eibach, R. P., & Gilovich, T. (2005). Here's looking at me: the effect of memory perspective on assessments of personal change. *Journal of Personality and Social Psychology, 88,* 50–62.

Ross, M., & Wilson, A. E. (2003). Autobiographical memory and conception of self: Getting better all the time. *Current Directions in Psychological Science, 12,* 66–69.

PHILIP G. ZIMBARDO, Stanford University

Saga of My Stealth Bomber Chapter: Can't Miss, But Vanished Without a Trace

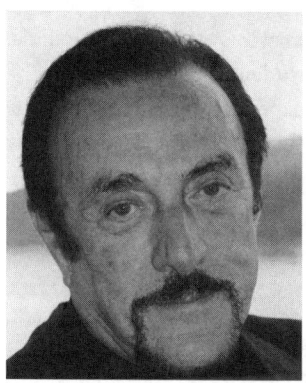

Before deciding to write a chapter covering decades of my research, I asked myself: What are the features, the academic criteria that should make it a can't-miss hit with my colleagues? I wanted it to be widely cited, to stimulate new research, to be viewed as a paradigm shift, and perhaps to spark a debate or two on the side. I needed to resurrect my career, which had been stuck in a basement dungeon of the Stanford Prison. I needed to go beyond just doing a dramatic demonstration to prove that I could also be a theorist, and a scholar as well.

So I would start with a new theory that generates a range of testable hypotheses, with a host of measurable behaviors. Then present a series of original experimental tests using novel and traditional methodologies. Throw in a set of case studies from a diverse body of literature that illustrates various aspects of the theory. Do the scholarly thing of including pithy quotes and hundreds of references that cut across many disciplines. Good to cite many colleagues so that they will feel the reciprocal obligation to cite back (a Cialdini influence extension). Also wonderful to be able to stretch out and develop these ideas with the broad brush stroke that writing a chapter allows, which most journal articles constrain. Finally, work with a good editor, and publish the chapter in a venue that is itself highly cited by my esteemed colleagues.

And I followed that script to the letter, starting with getting the lengthy chapter accepted in *Advances in Experimental Social Psychology* (Vol. 31, 1999), the most highly cited source for social psychologists. Mark Zanna was my esteemed editor, supporting this endeavor to the hilt, in fact with more enthusiasm than I had ever received since Mrs. Munvas gave me an A+ for my fifth-grade report on R. L. Stevenson's *Dr. Jekyll and Mr. Hyde*. How could I miss having covered every angle, with my 141-page chapter, brimming with over 280 references, nearly 20 quotes ranging from Milton, Pirandello, Emerson, Voltaire, Diderot, and Bertrand Russell to a Yiddish proverb tossed in for good measure? Did I mention the dozen detailed case studies from the obscure cause of Salem witchcraft to Freud's Anna O, to Cargo Cults, and my "miracle cure" of student suffering from multiple psychopathic symptoms?

Wait, I almost forgot the special ingredient that should generate a heated exchange in our field: Do a series of unethical experiments. In this case, the point of some of the research was to predict the onset of psychiatric symptoms of paranoia, phobia, and somatic disorders—by making normal student participants mad, for a short time. Of course, there would be extensive post-experimental debriefing, along with an original, extended discussion on research ethics under the heading: Why deception and distress may be necessary to study the "dark side of human nature." Diana Baumrind would surely be distressed enough to write an *American Psychologist* diatribe about unethical social psychologists like me since Stanley Milgram was no longer around to be hung out to dry.

Last but not least was a provocative title: "Discontinuity Theory: Cognitive and Social Searches for Rationality and Normality—May Lead to Madness." Sounds like Dissonance Theory, which was tops on the hit parade for decades; add in cognitive, social, and clinical psychology to the mix, with a dash of anthropology, and now surely it would be a chart buster. The theory was motivational and attributional at the same time as it was about self-processes. Am I covering all bases?

Here is the theory in a nutshell:

1. The perception of an experiential discontinuity—that is of personal relevance to one's self-concept—becomes a violation of expectation that triggers a powerful motivation to engage in one or more of the following actions.
2. To understand the cause of the discontinuity in order to appear rational to one's self and to others—generating a cognitive attributional search process.
3. To appear normal, to be comparable to others, despite the sense of a violation of expectation is being experienced—generating a social search process.
4. The need to suppress the overt arousal and deflect or ignore the experienced distress by direct actions—generating a behaviorally oriented search process.
5. These processes flow from the three most basic human needs: to know, to belong, to gain esteem.

6. After discussing the motivating effects of discontinuities and their many varieties, the theory makes specific predictions about behaviors that will flow from Actors focused exclusively on internal cognitive searches for rationality versus from Actors enmeshed in externally, situationally-centered social searches for normality.

7. Biased rationality notions lead to positing a set of learned explanatory frames utilized to account for a variety of discontinuities, such as body or health, the physical environment, or the social environment (people or groups), among others.

8. Now comes the hot stuff, when the theory predicts the links between particular kinds of explanatory biases and specific different emerging pathologies, both individual and psychiatric ones, and also social pathologies. Phobias will be dominant pathology only from those overusing physical environment attributions. Paranoia will be typical only from those relying on people-based explanatory search frames. Hypochondriasis, or somatoform disorders, will be the primary pathology generated only from those who explain their perceived discontinuities via reliance on body/health status. The social pathology equivalents are mass hysteria to hypochondriasis, as prejudice is to the individual pathology of paranoia, and vandalism is to phobia, and others that were described in the chapter.

The methodology and measures were both unusual and traditional: The special paradigm used hypnosis as the methodological tool to create controlled experiences of sudden discontinuities with or without explanation (Awareness vs. Amnesia) attributed to the hypnotic condition. Participants included those high and low in premeasured hypnotizability.

Among the many different outcomes measures used across the four experiments presented were: heart rate, respiration rate, EEG, EMG, Profile of Mood States, Subjective Units of Arousal, MMPI scales, Multiple Affect Adjective Checklist, TAT, sentence completions, Mood Adjective Check List, Emotion Circle, Profile of Mood States, Interpersonal Response Style, and other observational and behavioral indices. (See Zimbardo, LaBerge, & Butler, 1993, for psychophysiological measures of unexplained arousal.)

Across these different studies we were able to induce experienced partial deafness as a discontinuity that generated dramatic shifts toward paranoid thinking. In addition, we found high levels of physiological and emotional arousal with amnesia-based hypnotic inductions of basic changes in respiration and heart rate. Finally, and most dramatically, we found direct inductions of explanatory search frames of people, body/health, or physical environment in different experimental groups that lead to significant outcome measures of paranoia, somatoform disorders, and phobias as predicted by the explanatory attributional search processes that were experimentally induced in normal college students.

We even used clinical judgments of our participants by a dozen trained clinical psychologists in order to show that even they could not detect the basic normality of our participants as they were temporarily transformed into behaving and thinking in pathological ways.

Thus, we have a novel approach for understanding the onset of psychopathological symptoms in those with "pre-morbid" normality status. This should be of great relevance to clinical practice and theory. We are demonstrating that the most ordinary process of trying to make sense of a disharmony in one's experience can get side-railed into a biased search for meaning or the biased search to appear normal that generates irrational thinking and abnormal reactions. In every society, madness equals irrational plus abnormal in a given person.

Of course, by now you are intrigued to know about what the incredible predicted success was like once this chapter was published. It was a pebble dumped into a deep well, no sound coming back! To be accurate, a total of three colleagues informed me that they had read it, and found it interesting, one from Germany, another from Poland, along with a lone American. I treasure their e-mails and plan to frame them when I learn the art of framing better. I know of not a single citation to this chapter in the entire corpus of Western literature. My can't-miss *numero-uno* top-of-the-hit-parade chart buster—vanished somewhere between Stanford and the Bermuda Triangle. It never has surfaced again. I had laid it to rest until Bob Arkin forced me to relive this violation of my professional expectations, and to recite it shamefully to my esteemed colleagues, or at least the other 49 of the 50 losers represented in this volume.

WHAT IS MY TAKE ON THIS ABYSMAL FAILURE?

1. Nobody reads *Advances in Social Psychology*, they only raid the reference lists, or cite chapters that are in their mainstream. Graduate students can't afford its too-high price, so can only steal it from their faculty offices, which in recent years are now locked. [All volumes of *Advances in Experimental Social Psychology* are now available free, online, via Science Direct, if your university library has ordered the Science Direct version of the *Advances* series.]
2. It was too cognitive for social psychologists at that time, and too social for cognitive psychologists, and too clinical for both groups. Of course, the clinical psychologists who read the literature never read our *Advances*, only theirs.
3. Hypnosis is a strange and sinister phenomenon. Despite decades of solid research by Jack Hilgard and many others, including the venerable Clark Hull at Yale, it is rarely used as a methodology, or when it is it is given a nice-sounding name like "affect induction" instead of spooky stuff.
4. It was much too long. It was a short book that might have been a hit in paperback packaged with a Santana CD.
5. The title made it seem like it was all about "madness," which isn't scientific, and thus confusing why a smart guy like Mark Zanna would even decide to publish it.

I end my sad saga of this crash-and-burn flight of fancy with the hope that some-body out there will read it and tell me how to repackage it to revive it, and make it work as intended—or proclaim: Let it Rest In Peace.

There is one positive postscript to my story. One of our experiments was pub-lished in *Science* and got a very enthusiastic response from the scientific commu-nity, media, and advocates for the deaf (Zimbardo, Andersen, & Kabat, 1981). It was the study showing that unexplained partial deafness (in young hearing-able participants) led to strong paranoid reasoning, negative affect, and socially isolating behavior. Deafness in the elderly is often associated with the development of para-noia and institutionalization. My recommended cure when the first paranoid symp-toms surface in elderly family members, friends, or clients: buy a good hearing aid, and avoid any psychiatric misdiagnoses within costly, irrelevant therapy sessions.

REFERENCES

Zimbardo, P. G. (1981, December). The ethics of inducing paranoia in an experimental setting: A reply to M. Lewis, M.D. *IRB: A Review of Human Subjects Research*, 3, 1, 9, 10–11.

Zimbardo, P. G. (1999). Discontinuity theory: Cognitive and social searches for rationality and normality—may lead to madness. In M. P. Zanna (Ed.), *Advances in Experimental Social Psychology* (Vol. 31, pp. 345–486). San Diego, CA: Academic Press.

Zimbardo, P. G., Andersen, S. M., & Kabat, L. G. (1981, 26 June). Induced hearing deficit gen-erates experimental paranoia. *Science*, 212, 1529–1531.

Zimbardo, P. G., LaBerge, S., & Butler, L. (1993). Psychophysiological consequences of unex-plained arousal: A posthypnotic suggestion paradigm. *Journal of Abnormal Psychology*, 102, 466–473.

JENNIFER CROCKER, The Ohio State University

From Egosystem to Ecosystem

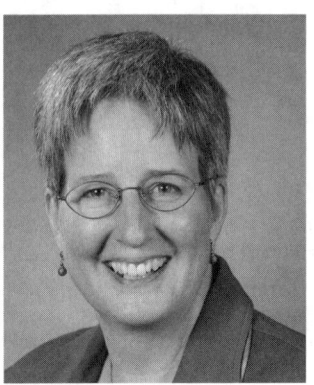

I am intrigued by the idea that many dissatisfactions in people's lives are things they actually created or at least contributed to. The power of this idea struck me when I attended a leadership development workshop conducted by Learning as Leadership (LaL). One take-away from the workshop was that, when things don't go the way they want, people usually view themselves as being at the mercy of other people and events. For example, when work is dissatisfying because we feel overwhelmed, or relationships are dissatisfying because relationship partners don't give us the support we want, we tend to feel somewhat victimized by the situation or other people. Yet, a little self-examination suggests that we actively participate in creating these experiences for ourselves. For example, when I feel overwhelmed it is usually because I agreed to too many requests, or procrastinated on a difficult project. When other people don't give me the support I want, it's often because I didn't express my need in a way that would elicit support, or I haven't been supportive of them. For a variety of reasons, we often find it difficult to see these connections between our own behavior and what we experience.

Understanding how and why people create what they don't want in their own lives and the lives of others could provide a powerful starting point for creating what they do want for themselves and others. As I experienced and observed at the workshop, this insight can make people more effective leaders, team members, and relationship partners. It's not enough, however, to know how we create what we don't want; we also need to understand how we can create what we do want for ourselves and others.

Paradoxically, I learned that people are most likely to create what they don't want when they have an egosystem perspective—when they focus on satisfying their own desires and needs to the exclusion of others'. In contrast, people are most likely to create what they do want when they have an ecosystem perspective—when they recognize that their own well-being cannot be separated from the well-being of others and the environment. Consequently, they focus on contributing to something larger than the self, such as the well-being of another person, project, or organization. These are not mutually exclusive possibilities—we can stop being driven by our egos and yet lack an ecosystem goal, or we can have an ecosystem goal, yet get caught up in our own egoistic desires.

This idea has proven very helpful to me in my own life, and I've seen that it is helpful to many people at the LaL workshops. Yet, I hadn't seen the power of this idea articulated in research on the self and social relationships. For the past 10 years, this has been my mission. The first part of the idea, that when we're driven by our egos we create what we don't want, was not terribly difficult to articulate, because a lot of social psychological research is consistent with this view. Lora Park and I organized much of this literature in a *Psychological Bulletin* paper on "The costly pursuit of self-esteem." That paper met with some resistance from social psychologists who believe that people need self-esteem and therefore need to pursue it. Nonetheless, it was a much easier sell than the most important part of the idea— that to a much larger degree than we realize, we have the power to create what we want in our lives. Specifically, when we take others' well-being into account, we often experience what we want for ourselves. Instead of being at the mercy of people and events, we can be "at the source," creating what we want by giving it away.

My collaborators and I operationalized this idea by studying two goals that epitomize these different approaches—self-image goals, which involve getting others to view the self in desired ways so we can get what we want, and compassionate goals, which involve being constructive and supportive of others. Most of my research on these goals examines how they play out in people's lives. In a series of daily and weekly report studies of individuals and roommate dyads, Amy Canevello, my graduate students, and I showed that on days or weeks students have compassionate goals, they give more support and are more responsive to others, and receive more support and responsiveness from others; feel more peaceful, clear, and connected; are less anxious and depressed; self-regulate better and make more progress toward their goals; and become more learning-oriented. When they have self-image goals, people neither give nor receive more support; they are less responsive and others are less responsive to them; they feel more afraid, confused, anxious, and depressed; they self-regulate worse; and they become more oriented toward validating themselves. Most of these effects hold when we examine effects on dependent variables the same day (or week), on lagged days (or weeks), and when we examine the effects of chronic goals (averaged across daily or weekly reports) on change in the dependent variable from pretest to posttest. Furthermore, over time as these experiences accumulate, they predict change in a range of beliefs about the self and relationships.

This idea and the data seem to elicit strong reactions, both favorable and unfavorable. On the positive side, our paper on the interactive effects of self-image and compassionate goals on changes in social support transactions was accepted at *JPSP* with only one round of reviews (Crocker & Canevello, 2008). On the negative side, papers articulating the theory, and effects of the goals on achievement goals, anxiety and depression, self-regulation, and growth (incremental) theories of relationships from the same data sets, all met with rejection.

Reviewers and editors have provided many justifications for their unfavorable responses. And naturally, I feel at the mercy of their judgments, which creates a sense of dissatisfaction. Some have complained that the predictions seem counterintuitive. And it is counter-intuitive that people are more likely to get what they want when they stop trying to get others to give it to them and start trying to give to others, and over time see that this can change beliefs. Upon reflection, however, it makes sense. For example, people with compassionate goals increase in growth beliefs about relationships, because when they have the goal to be compassionate and supportive of others, others respond, the relationship gets better, and therefore the belief that relationships can improve develops or strengthens. Editors and reviewers have described our findings as "odd," "implausible," and even "ludicrous," apparently because they run counter to conventional assumptions about the nature of goals, beliefs, and relationships.

Sometimes, reviewers and editors have suggested that the ideas and findings are nothing new. However, they differ wildly in what familiar effects they believe we have replicated. Reviewers and/or editors have variously suggested that the distinction between compassionate and self-image goals is simply (a) approach vs. avoidance, (b) intrinsic vs. extrinsic aspirations, (c) communion vs. agency, (d) negative vs. positive mood, (e) regulatory fit, (f) controlled vs. autonomous self-regulation, and (g) ego-involved or ability goals vs. learning or mastery goals. They have suggested that compassionate goals are the same thing as responsiveness, relationship quality, secure attachment, self-esteem, inclusion of others in the self, interdependence, and so on. Not surprisingly, the particular redundancy the reviewers detect depends on the dependent variable (and therefore, perhaps, the reviewer's specialization). It is difficult to believe that our measures of compassionate and self-image goals are strongly confounded with all of these constructs, and unparsimonious to assume that each effect of the goals is due to a different overlapping construct. Although we do not have data to rule out every alternative construct reviewers have mentioned, where we do have data none of the alternative constructs can account for the effects of compassionate and self-image goals.

The constructs of compassionate and self-image goals seem to function almost as projective tests, with people seeing in them their own preferred constructs. I'm not entirely sure why. Partly, I suspect, it's because to prepare manuscripts of manageable length and digestible findings, we have written up our results in different papers, focusing on mental health in one paper, self-regulation in another, social support in a third. Readers of one paper may be convinced they have identified the "true" construct that accounts for the effects of the goals, when that construct is implausible as an explanation of other findings. High on our priorities for future projects is a longer, *Advances*-type paper that provides a broad overview of the varied effects of the goals. Self-image and compassionate goals do, indeed, bear a "family resemblance" to a number of other constructs. Self-image goals resemble many "ego-involved" or self-esteem–oriented goals, although they focus in particular on controlling how others see the self. Compassionate goals resemble a number of constructs in social psychology, such as altruism, empathic concern, etc. But compassionate goals are not completely redundant with any of these constructs, and so far none of these other constructs fully accounts for the effects of compassionate goals.

Some reviewers have suggested that our papers need to include laboratory studies in which the goals are manipulated. We would love to include such studies. We are confident that we can manipulate self-image goals. However, manipulating compassionate goals is complex because the manipulation must induce caring about a specific target in a particular context. Consequently, a generic manipulation is unlikely to be effective. At the same time, social psychologists who hold up laboratory experiments as the gold standard of research methodology sometimes overestimate the strength of the causal inferences that can be drawn from experiments. For sure, if we hold everything constant except the thing we manipulate, we can conclude that something about the manipulation caused the observed effect. But all manipulations are imperfect operationalizations of constructs, and we often do not know with confidence what features of the manipulation account for its effect. Furthermore, daily and weekly report studies have a number of strengths that are usually lacking in laboratory experiments: they observe participants in vivo; they allow us to test change in same-day (or week), lagged-day (or week), and pretest-to-posttest analyses; and they allow us to examine upward and downward spirals that occur because effects are reciprocal—for example, self-image goals predict increased anxiety, and anxiety predicts increased self-image goals. These dynamic, reciprocal, and interpersonal effects are difficult, but not impossible, to study in the laboratory.

Although I sometimes feel frustrated by these responses and at the mercy of editors' and reviewers' judgments, I realize that focusing on how my research is underappreciated creates what I don't want—dissatisfaction, resentment, and competitive rather than supportive relations with others. Clarifying my compassionate goal, to do research that helps people create the lives they want, helps me to stop feeling at the mercy of reviewers and editors, and recognize that my frustration originates largely in my own struggle to define, operationalize, and explain concepts that LaL conveys experientially and ideographically. Each negative reaction illuminates a place where my thinking and writing could be clearer, or my research more compelling, for which (on my good days) I feel gratitude. Although my efforts have been imperfect, the data reinforce my belief that this work offers a useful perspective on the sources of dissatisfaction, and a powerful tool for change.

REFERENCE

Crocker, J., & Canevello, A. (2008). Creating and undermining social support in communal relationships: The role of compassionate and self-image goals. *Journal of Personality and Social Psychology, 95,* 555–575.

BERNARD WEINER, University of California, Los Angeles

Publish and Perish

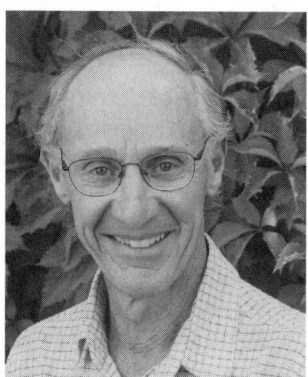

In earlier times, to ascend to one of the few available professorships at a European university, the candidate had to have a major publication, typically a lengthy book. Given the time such an undertaking required, and given the shorter lifespan in the past, not long after publication the author perished. This is the background for the phrase "publish and perish," which I would have liked to claim but honesty (and the fear of getting caught) did not allow.

But publish and perish can have an alternate meaning. The typical publication in psychology (and I imagine the other social and perhaps natural sciences as well) is rarely cited—that is, there is a sequence of publish and perish, although in this case the work rather than the author undergoes a demise. Surely most authors expect something other than this.

Regarding my personal history, I believe there is a fairly substantial correlation, say $r = 0.70$, between my view of the value of an article I have published and the importance or worth placed on it by the scientific community (operationalized as the number of received citations)—that is, the good articles are perceived as valuable and the poor articles are perceived as unworthy. There are any numbers of mechanisms responsible for this relation. It may be that my better articles are submitted to and published in the more prestigious (i.e., high citation impact) journals, where they are read and cited. Another possible explanation for the perceived relation between my personal judgments and the opinions of other psychologists is that I tend to place higher value on my theoretical than empirical articles. I suspect that theoretical works generate more interest and citations than do empirical studies (although this hypothesis is questioned, for example, by the citations generated by the Milgram obedience and Zimbardo prison research, which certainly are not highly theoretical). Finally, it may be that other psychologists see the world through the same lens as I do and we agree on what is important. I have to admit, however, that I doubt this (very much). Soon, I will return to the possibility of a lack of shared values when discussing a perceived underappreciated work.

Of course, a correlation of $r = 0.70$ also means that some articles I highly value are relatively dismissed by others, whereas some articles that I regard as less than significant seem to resonate with readers. Indeed, I have often found myself surprised when an article I do not consider strong is accepted on the initial submission, and/or later I find it highly cited. That also is a reasonable topic for a book, although I think most authors would prefer not to address this possibility (i.e., "Most over-appreciated …"). Given some over-evaluation of less-than-significant publications, any subsequent complaints I make regarding neglect are not sour grapes because I believe God already has evened the score.

But let me return to articles the author (me) thinks are of major importance yet they fail to have an impact on the psychological audience—that is, there is an instance of *publish and perish*. Again the reasons for this vary widely. There often is lack of agreement between reviewers, and perhaps an article I regard as significant is rejected on the basis of chance (choice of reviewers) and published in a so-called minor journal, where it does not receive attention. Or, perhaps I am misguided when judging the value of my own writings and others see a "poor" article for what it is worth. Authors are not good judges of their own works and churn out good and poor writings within close time frameworks that they fail to distinguish in regards to worth.

Finally, it also is possible that, for some unknown reasons, the readers fail to comprehend the value of a work that the author "correctly" regards as significant. History is filled with instances of, for example, published musical works from Bizet, Handel, and many others that listeners come to love only long after the death of the composer. Unfortunately, I doubt that this delayed reaction has been exhibited in the social sciences. I am not a historian of science, but I can't think of one psychological work that has made an impact only after an appreciable delay, say after the death of the author. Fritz Heider, my intellectual mentor in attribution theory, did experience an unusual lag between his initial writings and the acclaim of others, but even for Heider the delay period between his major book publication and recognition was about one decade, leaving him many years to bask in reflected glory. So for the writer of psychology, it is quite likely now or never (where "now" includes about a five-year time lag for the citing publications).

Let me, then, turn to one publication I feel has not received its just due and provide my attribution for the failure. This first requires some understanding of my personal history and the psychological Zeitgeist in the field of motivation when I began my graduate studies in 1959, more than 50 years ago (egad!).

PERSONAL GOALS

To understand the source of my psychological value system, I have to introduce my dissertation mentor, John W. Atkinson. For Atkinson, the goal for a motivational theorist is to systematically relate a set of constructs and bring them to bear on a variety of psychological phenomena. The goals of the Expectancy × Value theorists, which describes Atkinson, and for the Drive theorists such as Clark Hull and Kenneth Spence, were the same as those held by scientists in the physical sciences. It is indeed fair to state that, for Atkinson at least, Newton and Einstein were the guiding lights, with perhaps some limitations accepted because the subject matter of psychology was animate rather than inanimate objects so that individual differences between the objects had to be taken into account.

But aspirations and attainments are often discrepant. Atkinson's theory remained confined to the achievement domain, and even then his predictions often were not confirmed. The drive theorists suffered a similar fate of lack of generality and questionable hypotheses. By the 1960s, the so-called "grand" theories in motivation were on the decline, replaced by smaller, more focused models. These models were constrained to specific phenomena and sought for precise predictions within a narrow domain. But because I was trained in the milieu of the grand(iose) tradition in motivation, conceptual generalization and empirical breadth were ingrained as the aims toward which any respectable motivation theorist must strive. Of course, the usual theoretical tenets of parsimony, precision, and the like also were desired.

My work concerning achievement motivation initially followed in the Atkinson tradition but then moved to an attribution perspective. The focus first was on personal attributions following success and failure and their effects on subsequent motivation. But I also examined judgments and reactions following attributions for the failure of others. This naturally directed me to think about blame versus withholding blame for failure. Soon thereafter, rather than confining myself to achievement evaluation, I began to examine reactions to the stigmatized, help-giving, aggression, and other instances of social motivation where concepts such as fault, responsibility, and intention were applicable. I excitedly thought I was approaching the grandiose goal of creating a general theory of motivation. Although it was not in the Atkinsonian tradition of Expectancy × Value theory, it was consistent with the lofty goals of the motivation theorists of yore.

There came a time when there was sufficient literature, as well as new statistical techniques, to conduct a meta-analysis of two motivation domains that typically receive disparate theoretical treatments yet had both been addressed from an attributional perspective: help-giving and aggression. I thought if phenomena in these two areas could be explained with the same theory, a theory that had grown from the study of achievement striving, then a major step would have been taken toward the development of a unifying conception of motivation. I enlisted the aid of three colleagues who provided statistical expertise and they conducted the analyses as well as making other central contributions. The results were as satisfying as I could have desired: both supportive of attribution theory yet giving rise to some perplexing issues that would generate more research. For example, we found that helping is determined by attribution-generated emotion and could be represented as a sequence of uncontrollable need–sympathy–help-giving. For aggression, both the attribution and the emotion elicited by causal beliefs directly aroused action and could be depicted as a sequence of controllable act–anger–retaliation, where controllability also was proximally linked to the behavior. In sum, helping was a matter of only the heart whereas aggression was determined by both the head and the heart. But both altruism and aggression, as well as achievement evaluation, have causal beliefs and elicited emotions as their theoretical foundations.

I can't quite remember what happened next, which might be ascribed to age or to the more dynamic process of repression. I think we sequentially submitted a manuscript to two or three top journals, where it was rejected. We then sent a paper to *Cognition and Emotion*, which is a reasonable but not widely read outlet. An article was published (Rudolph, Roesch, Greitemeyer, & Weiner, 2004), and in the next five years it received 23 citations, which is above the median of article citations yet I regard as "near death." Of course, I am not willing to let it perish, and in a subsequent book (Weiner, 2006) I basically reproduced the published chapter and the meta-analyses tables. I also refer to the findings whenever I have the opportunity, which probably accounts for 25% of the article citations.

What do I think accounted for the lack of reader attention? I could attribute it to the lack of a popular outlet, but that still leaves me wondering why so many reviewers considered it unworthy of publication. My best guess is that my goal of theoretical generality, seeking to account for behavioral variance over a large domain of types of behavior, is not currently considered of high priority by others. That attribution theory predicts some help-giving and some aggression and some achievement with the same constructs does not raise any eyebrows. This lack of shared values is in part due to a Zeitgeist shift in the goal of motivational psychology away from the grand theories, a shift reflecting disagreements between generations as to what is important and what represents scientific progress. Of course, many other explanations are possible that perhaps make less use of a hedonic bias (e.g., this was not a "good" paper and was properly judged by the readers).

What advice, then, might I give to the next generation of research psychologists? First, it probably is the case that God evens the score: if you write and publish a great deal, sometimes you will come out popular when you should not and sometimes you will feel unfairly neglected. Withhold recrimination and blame when (not if) the latter occurs; just keep writing. Second, to your own self remain true—that is, decide on your personal scientific objectives and strive to accomplish them. In my example, striving includes repetition to make my point heard.

REFERENCES

Rudolph, U., Roesch, S. C., Greitemeyer, T., & Weiner, B. (2004). A meta-analytic review of help giving and aggression from an attributional perspective. *Cognition and Emotion, 18,* 815–848.

Weiner, B. (2006). *Social motivation, justice, and the moral emotions.* Mahway, NJ: Erlbaum Press.

ABRAHAM TESSER, University of Georgia, Emeritus

A Catastrophe in My Research Portfolio

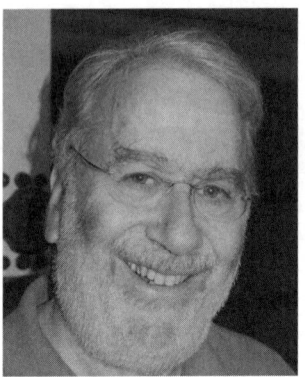

I am not sure why I agreed to write this essay. I don't do psychology anymore. And, as I look back on my psychology days I do not feel that my work was underappreciated. I used to read the journals and scholarly books regularly. If what I was reading had a title that was related to something that I had worked on, I would check to see if the author had referenced my work. I often thought they missed "my stuff." On the other hand, my work was cited often enough by others that I did not feel it was ignored. Later on I had an occasion to actually count references to the work of many, many social psychologists (Tesser & Bau, 2002). Although my work was never the "most cited," its place on the list was respectable. So, my work was, if anything, appreciated.

I find that extraordinary. I have an approach to knowledge that is not totally orthogonal but at least 45 degrees of separation from the approach of many others in the field. Many people believe that research is cumulative and self-corrective. As we abandon one theory for another in the light of empirical evidence we get closer to the "real" enduring "truth." Nature will reveal her ultimate secrets (i.e., "Truth") if we simply collect enough data. I don't believe this.

Like many philosophers of science, in my heart of hearts I do not believe that there is a scientific "Truth." And, data, by itself, reveal nothing. Data are merely a way to keep score in judging the utility of a theory or hypothesis. The theory or hypothesis is never True, but some are better (either in breadth or precision) at anticipating actual experience (i.e., data) than others. Dem's the rules of the game. And, to be sure, from my perspective, it is much more a game than a search for truth.

Many are in social psychology because they want to make a difference. They want to increase fairness for women, gays, racial minorities. They want to decrease depression and increase self-esteem; they want to engender happiness; they want to decrease aggression; they want to improve the quality of intimate relationships. These are all, more or less, noble goals, but that isn't what drove me as a psychologist.

I spent decades enthusiastically pursuing research in social psychology. I did not do it for the money. (Although, if the truth be known, the money was good, not Wall Street bonus good but good enough.) I wasn't driven because I thought that I was moving the field closer to Truth, and I wasn't driven because I thought the world would be a better place because of my work.

What drove me as a psychologist, and what drives me now as a furniture maker, is the esthetic of the idea underlying the work. I just like contemplating ideas that are novel, surprising, simple (but not too simple), integrative, and upsetting. I have written a bit about such ideas, which I call S ideas, and contrasted them with Boring or B ideas (Tesser, 2000). Of course, any idea, whether it be an S idea or a B idea, that happens to be competing in a scientific realm must anticipate and organize data to be useful. The greater the accuracy of its predictions and the broader the domain of its application, then the more useful is the idea.

All of this brings me to the catastrophe in my research portfolio. I am a fan of formal models. In the 1970s a French mathematician by the name of René Thom began exploring and describing a topographical model intended to model dynamical systems. The systems he described were sometimes stable and other times unstable. The behavior of the system sometimes showed large, discontinuous, dramatic (or catastrophic) changes. Thom called his system "catastrophe theory." (Similar, more current views of these nonlinear dynamics have been captured and popularized by Malcom Gladwell in *The Tipping Point* [2000]). Catastrophe theory captured my interest immediately. When applied to certain social behavior it seemed to provide a succinct way of describing many important phenomena. The description made intuitive sense and, as an added bonus, it did so in a way that flouted several usual assumptions underlying more paradigmatic research.

I will try to illustrate this with an example (Tesser, 1980). Suppose we want to understand the intimacy of A's behavior toward B. Let us make the plausible assumption that such behavior is a function of A's personal disposition toward B (i.e., how much he likes her). The more he likes her, the more intimate his behavior toward her. Let us also assume that there may be social pressure working in the opposite direction (e.g., norms against dating a person from her ethnic group, a large disparity in age or social class, etc.). The greater the social pressure against intimacy with B the less A's intimate behavior.

We usually think of changes in behavior as being proportional to, or a relatively smooth function of, changes in relevant circumstances. One might write a regression equation with an index of liking and an index of counter-pressure as predictors. Intimacy would be predicted to be a smooth, additive function of both parameters. But catastrophe theory suggests another set of plausible possibilities. Suppose social pressure is very high: B is from the wrong ethnic group, is the wrong age, has a criminal record, etc. Under theses circumstances we would not be surprised that as A goes from minimal liking, to moderate, to even moderately high liking, overt intimacy remains low and shows almost no change. Why would A risk social sanctions for someone he is not "crazy" about? At some point, however, at a high level of liking, even a small increment in B's attractiveness will cause A to suddenly show a large, disproportionate jump to high levels of intimacy. Dissonance theory suggests that when the jump from low to high intimacy comes, intimacy will be even more pronounced *because of* the strong, dissonant social pressure. I think such discontinuities in affective behavior (e.g., intimacy, aggression) are not uncommon, particularly where social pressure is high.

Social pressure against B is still strong. Now let's go in the other direction. This time A starts out crazy about B and in a very intimate relationship with her. A finds out some things about B that decrease his attraction to her. As his attraction to B decreases, will his behavior toward her follow the same curve described above? Catastrophe theory suggests that it will not; A will continue at high levels of intimacy even as his liking decreases beyond the point where he suddenly jumped toward greater intimacy (in the paragraph above)—that is, he will continue showing intimate behaviors even as liking decreases beyond the point that caused the upward jump in intimacy. The psychology of this prediction seems right. Both commitment theory and dissonance theory suggest that it is more difficult to let go of something for which you have suffered (i.e., risked social ostracism). Of course, if attraction continues to go down, there will be a point at which intimacy declines and the catastrophe theory model suggests that intimacy will decline precipitously.

Catastrophe theory is different from the regression approach in yet another way. When social pressure is high and liking is moderately high the regression model predicts *a single behavior*: an additive combination of liking and social pressure. Catastrophe theory makes a different prediction. Some people are showing high levels of intimacy (those whose liking is decreasing) while others are showing little to no intimacy (those whose liking is increasing but have not yet crossed the threshold). The catastrophe prediction is *bimodality* under these circumstances while the regression prediction is univocal, moderate intimacy.

The model also has a place for smooth, proportional changes in behavior. If there is little social pressure in opposition to an intimate relationship with B, then the theory agrees with the regression model. It predicts that intimacy will be a smooth, proportional function of liking. Increases in liking will be reflected in proportional increases in intimacy; decreases in liking will be reflected in decreases in intimacy. Any particular level of liking will be reflected in the same level of intimacy regardless of whether that level of liking reflects an increase or a decrease.

I found looking at the conflict between internal dispositions and social constraints through the lens of catastrophe theory to be delightful. It was integrative: It had elements of dissonance theory, commitment theory, order effects, threshold phenomena, and person × situation interactions. It was systemic: All of these elements worked together in a system. It was heuristic, suggesting a new way at looking at this classic conflict.

I loved this model. I published it. It went nowhere. Was it underappreciated? Not at all. I loved this model for its novelty, its beauty, its "S"-ence. Regrettably, I could not pair it with convincing sets of data. For a scientific idea to be useful it must, ultimately, anticipate measurable, replicable experience. Dem's the rules of the game. And, in spite of my penchant for the esthetic, I too play the game by the rules.

So, what, if anything, is to be learned from this tale? First, there is beauty in science. Second, pursuing beauty in science is as legitimate and as scientifically productive a goal as trying to improve society. Finally, according to Keats (1819), "Beauty is truth, truth beauty." There are many ways of apprehending the world and Keats may be quite right with respect to some, but for science, "It ain't necessarily so."

REFERENCES

Gladwell, M. (2000). *The tipping point: How little things can make a big difference*. New York: Little Brown.

Keats, J. (1819/1884). Ode to a Grecian urn. In F. T. Palgrave (Ed.), *The poetical works of John Keats*. London: Macmillan.

Tesser, A. (1980). When individual dispositions and social pressure conflict: A catastrophe. *Human Relations, 33,* 393–407.

Tesser, A. (2000). Theories and hypotheses. In R. Sternberg (Ed.), *Guide to publishing in psychology journals* (pp. 58–80). Cambridge, UK: Cambridge University Press.

Tesser, A., & Bau, J. J. (2002). Social psychology: Who we are and what we do. *Personality and Social Psychology Review, 6,* 72–85.

DAN P. McADAMS, Northwestern University

I Want to Be a Social Psychologist

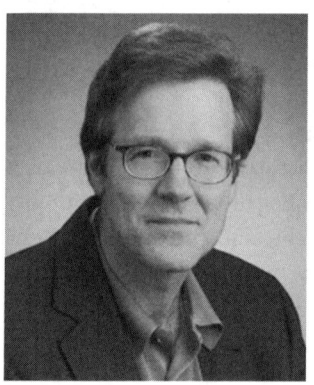

You may be wondering: *What is this guy doing in the book?*

Good question! I confess that I am not a social psychologist, at least not by conventional definitions. Whenever I've managed to sneak an article past the editors of *JPSP*, it has landed in that third section, on personality processes and individual differences. But I have tried to be a social psychologist, I swear! I have tried at least three times. But I keep getting the cold shoulder.

My choice for the most underappreciated "gem" in my work is a paper, now in its third incarnation, that has never actually been published. It keeps getting rejected by social psychologists! And because *it* (the paper) is an extension of *me*, I know that *I* have been rejected. (Being asked, therefore, to write a piece for this volume on social psychologists is some kind of dissonance task that I can't quite work through yet.)

My sad story begins in Orono, Maine, in the summer of 1992. Social psychologists and scholars in family studies and communications gathered together at the University of Maine for an international conference on personal relationships. Because my early research on intimacy motivation was enjoying some recognition at the time, I was asked to give one of the keynote addresses for the conference. The conference organizers did not know, however, that I was no longer professionally invested in the topic of intimacy. By the early 1990s, I had shifted focus to what has become my main contribution in psychology—the study of the life story, or *narrative identity*, and its role in the structure and the development of personality (and self). I should have told the organizers that I wasn't doing intimacy anymore. But I was young, and confident that I could put together something that the social psychologists would like.

The name of my talk was "How the *I* and the *Me* Come To Be: Attachment versus Intimacy." I think it's a nice title, don't you? I like that little rhyme in the first half, and the second half promises that my talk will be relevant to the conference theme—personal relationships. Reading the text over this morning, 18 years later, I admit there are more than a few problems. And it is all way too abstract for a conference on personal relationships. Still, I love this talk! Going back to William James's (1892/1963) distinction between the self as subject (the I) and the self as object (the Me), I first spelled out how the "I" is a *process* of meaning-making (subjectively construing and appropriating conscious experience as "mine") whereas the "Me" is the *product* of that process (the self that is made, variously called a self-concept, self-identity, and so on). Second, I sharpened the distinction between attachment (as a bond of protective love that forms in the first year of life between infant and caregiver) and intimacy (as a reciprocal experience of sharing and disclosure between two more-or-less mature individuals). Third (and this is the best part), I argued that the self-as-I *emerges* in the context of an evolving attachment relationship in the first two years of life, whereas the self-as-Me is *constructed* later on in life as a function (in part) of intimate relationships. In some deep psychological sense that was apparent to me (and apparently only me) at the time, attachment is to the I what intimacy is to the Me.

The audience was kind enough to applaud when my talk was finished, but I knew it had not gone over well. I don't recall what questions I got, if any, at the end, but I remember that I was shunned for the remainder of the conference. Well, that is too strong: People were friendly enough, but nobody seemed to want to talk about my talk, even though there was plenty of conversation about the other papers and presentations at the conference. There was also some sort of dancing party in the evening following my address, and I remember asking two different women (both social psychologists) to dance, and they both turned me down. I am sure they hated my talk.

A few years later, I dusted off the text from the Orono presentation and decided to rework it into a theoretical paper for *Personality and Social Psychology Review*. *PSPR* was a relatively new journal back then, and (as I recall it now) the editorial staff had recently sent out earnest appeals for new and creative papers. They seemed desperate. My new paper went beyond the Orono talk to introduce two more distinctions. The first is between (1) *self-concept* as a more-or-less generic term for what William James meant by the Me and (2) *identity*, which is the particular form the self-concept (the Me) takes in young adulthood when it becomes organized into a psychosocial structure that provides adult life with some degree of unity and purpose. (This way of thinking about identity as an emerging-adulthood structure that aims to provide life with unity and purpose ultimately traces back to Erik Erikson, but we don't have time to go there now.)

The second distinction refers to two different ways that self-concepts get made into identities—that is, two different ways that the I (in young adulthood and beyond) strives to make the Me into an identity. The first way follows what Jerome Bruner (1986) described as the *paradigmatic* approach to knowing, whereby the I tries to organize the semantic information of the self-concept into a theory about the self. The second is when the I takes what Bruner called the *narrative* route, working like an author or novelist to put episodic information of the self-concept together into an integrative story. Put simply, the I may be a theorist (paradigmatic) or an author (narrative), a Darwin or a Dostoyevsky. My own work suggests that most of us are more like Dostoyevsky much of the time. We try to make our lives into stories. My revised argument, therefore, linked my early work on intimacy to my emerging understanding of identity as a life story.

Knowing that I would need to win over social psychologists in order to get this paper published in *PSPR*, I read many articles and books regarding how social psychologists think about the self. I sent the paper out to two senior social psychologists whom I greatly admired. I should have known there was trouble, however, when neither of them wrote back. My response from the editor at *PSPR* was a flat-out rejection. The reviewers said that the paper was trying to do too many things. They also suggested that they did not like any of the things it was trying to do. They insisted that the concepts of attachment and intimacy were more similar than different, and they could see no merit whatsoever in all the theoretical musings about the I and the Me. On this latter point, my wife completely agrees. Whenever I feel the urge to wax passionate about the I and the Me with friends or at a party (this happens a lot), she quickly changes the subject.

My spirit broken after two rejections from social psychologists, I put these ideas away for a number of years while I did more productive things. For the next decade or so, I focused much of my attention on the psychological and cultural meanings of the life stories (narrative identities) constructed by especially generative and mature mid-life American adults. The central theme in many of these stories is *redemption*, or the deliverance from suffering to an enhanced status or state (McAdams, 2006).

Like Freud's "return of the repressed," however, my Orono ideas found their way back into my consciousness a couple of years ago. Invited to write a broadly integrative chapter on self and identity for a handbook of lifespan development, I found myself once again obsessed with the distinction between I and Me and challenged again to read the social-psychological literature on self, along with treatments of the topic in personality and developmental psychology, cognitive science, sociology, and the humanities. My new scheme built on certain other ideas developed in my research on redemptive life narratives to envision the self now as developing in three psychological layers. The I begins as a social *actor*, as the Me comes to encompass characteristic social roles and temperament traits. In mid-childhood, a second layer begins to form—the I as a motivated *agent*, conferring upon the Me personal goals, values, and strategies. In young adulthood, the I finally becomes an autobiographical *author*, as the Me takes on qualities of an integrative story of self.

The new synthesis (McAdams & Cox, 2010) successfully reframes some of the original ideas in the Orono paper, but it leaves others (like what to do with attachment and intimacy) still hanging. In search of redemption, I am now about to launch a third effort to win favor with social psychologists, as I rework the argument for a review paper that connects more explicitly to social-psychological conceptions of self and identity. With this all in mind, I recently worked up the nerve to send the lifespan development chapter to a valued colleague in social psychology. (I will not say if he is one of the 50 social psychologists in this book.) I asked if he might look parts of the chapter over and send along advice for my effort to develop the ideas further. He wrote back and said that he disliked my first sentence so much that he could not bring himself to read any further. This is true.

What lessons may be drawn from my story? Despite my colleague's discouraging response, I am resolved to write something that makes some good use of the ideas I introduced in Orono for a social psychology audience. Like a moth to the flame, I am still trying to be accepted by social psychologists! Now, part of my story is tongue-in-cheek, of course. I have made myself sound somewhat more pathetic and paranoid than I probably am, and I have doubtlessly exaggerated the negative responses from social psychologists. We all should know, furthermore, that acceptance by one's peers is not the be-all-and-end-all in our profession. I do believe that a scientist or scholar should pursue his or her best ideas with passion, even in the face of criticism or (worse) benign neglect. But there is also value and truth in the striving for acceptance, for it is the community of scientists and scholars with whom we work that ultimately determines (today or tomorrow) the credibility and utility of our ideas and our findings. Our model for our work, therefore, is *not* the mad scientist who works in isolation—the beautiful mind who is incomprehensible to others. Social psychologists know better than anybody else that we are social animals, sharing ideas and learning from each other. Science is (broadly construed) a social enterprise.

But science is also a deeply personal enterprise. With that in mind, what I like best about my long struggle to be accepted by social psychologists is the way it keeps bringing me back to an unfinished intellectual project, a kind of conceptual Zeigarnik effect for me. Okay, I am still a little bit annoyed that those two young social psychologists wouldn't dance with me in Orono, Maine. But (evolutionary psychology notwithstanding) what largely drives me back to the underappreciated and half-baked ideas that I expressed at that conference is the deep desire *to get it right*. Of course, none of us ever gets it totally right. Still, we keep working on our own intellectual projects, editing old ideas and combining them with new ones, incorporating new findings into old frameworks or changing those frameworks as new findings show them to be wanting, appropriating what we experience as scientists and as human beings into a lifelong intellectual obsession. Even in the face of rejection, there is a kind of ongoing redemption in it all, as nascent ideas grow into better concepts over the long haul.

Therefore, I am sticking with my most underappreciated gem. You social psychologists beware! Someday ...

REFERENCES

Bruner, J. S. (1986). *Actual minds, possible worlds.* Cambridge, MA: Harvard University Press.
James, W. (1892/1963). *Psychology.* Greenwich, CT: Fawcett.
McAdams, D. P. (2006). *The redemptive self: Stories Americans live by.* New York: Oxford University Press.
McAdams, D. P., & Cox, K. (2010). Self and identity across the lifespan. In A. Freund, & R. Lerner (Eds.), *Handbook of lifespan development:* Vol. 2 (pp. 158-207). New York: Wiley.

ALBERT BANDURA, Stanford University

But What About that Gigantic Elephant in the Room?

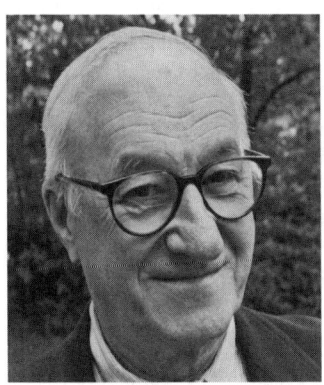

When I began my career, more than half a century ago, behaviorism had a stranglehold on the field of psychology. It focused almost entirely on learning by direct experiences through paired stimulation and response consequences. This type of theorizing was at odds with the conspicuous social reality that much of what people learn is through the power of social modeling. Direct experience is an unmercifully tough teacher. Hence, people shortcut the tedious, costly, and potentially hazardous process of trial and error by observational learning from the myriad modeling influences in their social and symbolic environment.

BELIEVING CAN BE BLINDING

Early in the behaviorist era, Watson and Thorndike proclaimed the non-existence of observational learning with a few cursory animal studies. It did not stop puppies from learning by observation novel ways of securing rewards, or chimpanzees raised in a human household from dressing up, applying lipstick, and prying lids off cans with screwdrivers. In the more contemporary theorizing, Skinnerians converted social modeling to a conditioned reinforcer. Hullian theorists recast modeling as simply a special case of discrimination learning. A model provides a social cue, the observer performs a matching response, and its reinforcement strengthens matching behavior.

It was in this inhospitable conceptual climate that I launched a program of research on the determinants of observational learning and the mechanisms through which it operates. In the conceptual scheme informing this research, social modeling through observational learning was governed by four constituent processes (Bandura, 1986). Attentional processes determine what is selectively observed in the profusion of modeling influences and what information is extracted from ongoing modeled events. People cannot be much influenced by observed events if they do not remember them. Through representational processes the information conveyed by modeling influences is converted to memory codes. Translational processes come into play in turning symbolic conceptions into appropriate courses of action. Motivational processes regulate whether people act on what they have learned observationally.

Diverse lines of research testified to the centrality and pervasiveness of observational learning and added to our understanding of how it works. Social cognitive theory also broadened the scope of the effects of social modeling and the functions it serves. In addition to promoting cognitive and behavioral competencies, modeling influences were shown to alter motivation; create and modify emotional proclivities; serve as social prompts that activate, channel, and support given styles of behavior; and shape images of reality.

Social modeling was gaining recognition, but there were a number of entrenched misconceptions about it that put a damper on research on this powerful mode of learning and social influence. They had to be laid to rest. One such misconception was that modeling, construed as "imitation," could produce only response mimicry. The caricature of social modeling as "monkey see/monkey do" is mistaken monkey business. In fact, most modeling is generative rather than superficial mimicry. Exemplars usually differ in content and other details but embody the same underlying principle. For example, the passive linguistic form may be embodied in any variety of utterances. Modeling involves abstracting the information conveyed by specific exemplars about the structure and the underlying principles governing the behavior rather than simply mimicking the specific exemplars. In abstract modeling, it is generative rules rather than particular exemplars that are being learned from the modeled information. Once individuals learn the guiding principle, they can use it to generate new versions of the behavior that go beyond what they have seen and heard.

Another oft-repeated misconception concerns the scope of modeling. Many activities involve cognitive skills on how to acquire and use information for predicting and solving problems. Critics argued that modeling cannot build cognitive skills because thought processes are covert and are not adequately reflected in modeled actions, which are the end-products of the cognitive operations. This was a limitation of conceptual vision rather than an inherent limitation of modeling. Cognitive skills can be made observable and are effectively cultivated by cognitive modeling. In this approach, models verbalize aloud their reasoning strategies and cognitive self-management of motivation and affective reactions as they engage in problem-solving activities.

Another misconception requiring retirement claimed that modeling is antithetical to creativity. Quite the contrary. There are several ways in which modeling promotes innovativeness. Modeling novel ways of thinking and doing things fosters innovativeness in others, whereas modeling conventional styles curtails it. When exposed to diversity in modeling, individuals usually do not pattern their behavior solely after a single model. Rather, they combine various aspects of different models into new blends of characteristics that differ from the original sources. Through the process of selective hybridization, diversity of modeling can spawn emergent novelty. It should also be noted that intended innovations are rarely entirely new. Rather, creativeness usually involves synthesizing existing knowledge into new ways of thinking and doing things. Innovators select useful elements from different exemplars, improve upon them, synthesize them into new forms, and tailor them to their particular pursuits. In these diverse ways, selective modeling serves as the mother of innovation.

There is still another well-entrenched misconception that requires correction. This concerns the oft-cited Bobo doll experiment on the transmission of novel forms of aggression through social modeling. Diverse lines of research identified four separable classes of effects of exposure to modeled aggression. It can teach novel aggressive styles of conduct; weaken restraints over interpersonal aggression by legitimizing, glamorizing, and trivializing violent conduct; desensitize and habituate viewers to human cruelty; and shape public images of reality by how it represents social and power relations and the norms and structure of societies. Clarification of each of these separable effects requires a different methodology.

The mistaken critique, which continues to be repeated in our textbooks, is that the study used a non-human target and Bobo dolls are for punching. The Bobo doll laboratory experiments were designed to clarify *observational learning*. The methodology for measuring learning effects requires conditions in which viewers feel free to reveal all they have learned. In the case of aggression, this requires simulated targets rather than retaliative ones. To use human targets to assess the instructive function of televised influence would be as nonsensical as to require bombardiers to bomb San Francisco, New York, or some other inhabited locations to test their level of acquisition of bombing skills.

We were not interested in whether children punched the Bobo doll. Rather, we measured whether children assaulted it in the novel modeled ways, such as pummeling it with a mallet and voicing the novel aggressive neologisms as they assaulted the doll. Children in the central condition never exhibited the novel forms of aggression. Although modeled aggression was only one among a variety of experimental methods we used to clarify the mechanisms governing observational learning, it is the only one that is featured in portrayals of social cognitive theory.

Our major theories of human behavior were formulated long before the revolutionary advances in communication technologies. A growing influential source of social learning is the pervasive symbolic modeling in the cyberworld through the electronic media. Unlike learning by doing, which requires altering the actions of each individual through repeated trial-and-error experiences, symbolic modeling can transmit information of virtually limitless variety to vast populations simultaneously in widely dispersed locales. The electronic era is transforming the nature, reach, speed, and loci of human influence (Bandura, 2002). Life in the cyberworld is enhancing the primacy and reach of symbolic modeling. Modeled new ideas, values, and styles of behavior are now being rapidly spread worldwide in ways that foster a globally distributed consciousness.

A DOSE OF AGENCY FOR THE REDUCTIONISTIC REVIVAL

Social cognitive theory is founded on an agentic perspective toward human self-development, adaption, and change (Bandura, 2006a). To be an agent is to influence the course of events by one's action. In this view, people are contributors to their life circumstances, not just products of them. Personal agency operates within a broad network of sociostructural influences. In these agentic transactions, people create social systems and the practices of social systems, in turn, influence how people live their lives.

The exercise of human agency is dismissed by physical eliminationists on the grounds that human behavior is regulated by neuronal mechanisms operating at a subpersonal level outside of one's awareness and control. Deliberative, reflective, self-referential, and other high-level cognitive events are dismissed as epiphenomenal events that create an illusion of control but actually have no effect on how one behaves. In this view, humans are essentially conscious hosts of automata that dictate their behavior subpersonally.

Proponents of this view frame the issue of personal regulation in the wrong terms at the wrong level of control. In acting as agents, individuals obviously are neither aware of, nor directly control their neuronal mechanisms. Rather, they exercise second-order control. They do so by intentionally engaging in activities at the macrobehavioral level known to promote given types of outcomes. In pursuing these activities, over which they can exercise control, they shape the functional circuitry and enlist the neurophysiological events subserving their pursuits. To use an analogy, in driving an automobile to a desired place, the driver engages in coordinated acts of shifting gears, steering, manipulating the gas pedal, and applying brakes. These deliberate acts, which the driver controls directly, regulate the mechanical machinery to get safely to where the driver wants to go. But the driver has neither awareness nor understanding of the correlative microcombustion, transmission, and braking processes subserving the driver's purposes. The deliberate planning of where to go on a trip, what route to take, what to do when one gets there, and securing reservations for these diverse activities far in advance requires considerable proactive top-down cognitive regulation. The internal combustion engine is the subserver, not the deliberative agent of the trip.

Each level of complexity—atomic, molecular, biological, psychological, and social structural—involves emergent new properties that are distinct to that level and, therefore, must be explained in its own right. For example, knowing the locality and brain circuitry subserving learning can say little about how best to motivate people to attend to, process, and organize relevant information, and whether learning is better achieved independently, cooperatively, or competitively. The optimal conditions must be specified by psychological principles. There is little at the subatomic or neuronal level that can tell us how to develop efficacious parents, teachers, and social reformers or how to build and run social systems.

The sensory, motor, and cerebral systems are tools people use to accomplish the tasks and goals that give meaning, direction, and satisfaction to their lives (Bandura, 2008; Harre & Gillet, 1994). An aspiring pianist, for example, has to practice tenaciously to train the brain, build muscular strength and dexterity, and hone sensory acuity to realize a virtuoso performance. It is not as though the neural network is really the pianist and the indefatigable musician is just a self-aggrandizing illusionist.

ADDRESSING CONTENTIOUS DUALISMS

Contentious dualisms pervade our field pitting individualism against collectivism, autonomy against interdependence, agency against communion, and social structure against personal agency. Among these dualities, the construal of individualism and collectivism as monolithic cultural traits is especially prevalent in our field. Sometimes they come with biased positive and negative attributed values.

Cultures are dynamic and internally diverse systems, not static monoliths. The categorical approach masks extensive intracultural diversity and important differences in cultures assigned to the same category. Not only are cultures not monolithic entities, but they are no longer insular. A variety of social forces, including transnational interdependencies, global market forces, and the growing primacy of cyberworld in people's lives worldwide, is homogenizing some aspects of life, polarizing other aspects, and fostering a lot of cultural hybridization.

It is widely claimed that Western theories lack generalizability to non-Western cultures. One must distinguish between basic human capacities and how culture shapes these potentialities into diverse forms. For example, social modeling is essential for self-development and functioning regardless of the culture in which one resides. Modeling is a universalized human capacity. But what is modeled, how modeling influences are structured, and the purposes it serves varies in different cultural milieus.

The same distinction in levels of analysis applies to perceived efficacy. A common duality misconstrues self-efficacy as self-centered aggrandizement of an autonomous self and contrasted with an interdependent communal one. Self-efficacy does not come in only an individualistic form, nor with a built-in value system. People's belief in their efficacy is exercised in individual, proxy, and collective forms. Social cognitive theory is, therefore, just as relevant to human attainments realized through interdependent collective effort as to those achieved individually. The relative weight given to individual, proxy, and collective modes of agency in the agentic blend may vary cross-culturally, but all agentic modes are needed to make it through the day wherever one lives.

In the agency/communion duality, agency is often negatively portrayed as the egocentric exercise of power and personal domination, whereas communion is benignly characterized as socially caring and oriented toward the common good. In point of fact, the agentic exercise of efficacy can serve communal purposes, and collectiveness can be stifling and oppressive.

Being immobilized by self-doubt about one's capabilities and belief in the futility of effort has little adaptive advantage. A growing body of research shows that, indeed, a resilient sense of efficacy has generalized functional value regardless of whether one resides in an individualistically oriented culture or collectivistically oriented one (Bandura, 2002). But how efficacy beliefs are developed, the form they take, the ways in which they are exercised, and the purposes to which they are put vary cross-culturally. The cross-cultural findings debunk the misconception that belief in one's efficacy is an egocentric orientation wedded to Western individualism.

In short, there is a cultural commonality in basic agentic capacities and mechanisms of operation, but diversity in the culturing of these inherent capacities. In this dual-level analysis, universality is not incompatible with manifest cultural plurality. Cultural variations emerge from universalized capacities through the influence of social practices reflecting shared values and norms, incentive systems, role prescriptions, and pervasive modeling of distinctive styles of thinking and behaving.

GOING GLOBAL WITH SOCIAL COGNITIVE THEORY

The value of a theory in the social sciences is judged by three criteria: explanatory, predictive, and operative power. Explanation is the easiest criterion to fulfill because one can devise a coherent scheme to account for events after the fact. Prediction is a tougher criterion, but one can foretell events without knowing why they occur. Theory-derived predictions are more informative, however. The value of a theory is ultimately judged by its power to provide reliable guides for effecting change. If aeronautical scientists developed aerodynamic theories but could never build an aircraft that can fly, their theorizing would not be taken seriously.

Global applications of social cognitive theory to promote society-wide changes testify to its efficacy to improve the quality of life in diverse cultural milieus (Bandura, 2006b). These applications, which reach millions of people in Africa, Asia, and Latin America, address some of the more urgent global problems. Using long-running serialized dramas as the vehicle for personal and social change, this model helps people to see a better life and informs, enables, and motivates them to take the steps to realize it. The generic principles are generalizable to diverse cultures with functional adoptions tailored to particular cultural values and social conditions. Worldwide applications of this model are raising national literacy, enhancing the status of women in societies in which they are marginalized and denied their liberty and dignity, reducing unplanned childbearing that perpetuates the cycle of poverty, curtailing the spread of the AIDS epidemic, promoting environmental conservation practices, and in other ways bettering people's lives. Tell the millions of people worldwide who have improved their lives that the type of theory guiding this effort is a self-centered Western theory that is not generalizable to non-Western cultures.

SHUNNING THE FORTUITOUS ASPECT OF LIFE

There is much that people do planfully to exercise some measure of control over their self-development and life circumstances. But there is a lot of fortuity in the courses lives take. Indeed, some of the most important determinants of life paths occur through the most trivial circumstances (Bandura, 1982; Merton & Barber, 2004). People are often initiated into new life trajectories, marital partnerships, and occupational careers through fortuitous circumstances. To cite an example, an academic publisher entered the lecture hall as it was rapidly filling up and seized an empty chair near the entrance. Some months later, he marries the woman who happened to be seated next to him. With only a momentary change in time of entry, seating constellations would have altered and this intersection would not have occurred. A marital partnership was thus fortuitously formed at a talk devoted to fortuitous determinants of life paths! As this event illustrates, a seemingly insignificant fortuitous event can set in motion concatenating influences that change life courses, that cascade toward an outcome that could not have been anticipated.

Fortuitous intersects introduce probabilistic uncertainties that complicate long-range predictions of human behavior. The physical sciences acknowledge indeterminacy at the quantum mechanical level in the physical world. Fortuitous events introduce an element of indeterminacy in the behavioral sciences. However, the field of psychology avoids chance like the plague. We are in the business of explaining, predicting, and modifying behavior. Chance is a troublesome nuisance that is simply ignored. We need to bring science to bear on the fortuitous aspect of life.

Most fortuitous events leave people untouched, others have some lasting effects, and still others branch people into new trajectories of life. Psychology does not have much to say about the occurrence of fortuitous intersects except, at the population level, the types of settings in which one moves, and the types of people who populate those settings make some types of intersects more probable than others: Hanging out in a university library will spawn different intersects than hanging out with the Hell's Angels. However, psychology can provide the basis for predicting the nature, scope, and strength of impact that fortuitous events will have on people's lives. In a first excursion into a predictive conceptual scheme (Bandura, 1982), social cognitive theory specifies how key personal attributes work in concert with inviting environmental properties to shape the course of events set in motion by fortuitous events.

Fortuitous events may be unforeseeable, but fortuity does not mean uncontrollability of its effects. Paradoxically, people can bring personal influence to bear on the fortuitous character of life (Bandura, 1998). They can make chance happen by pursuing an active life that increases the number and type of fortuitous encounters they will experience. Chance favors the inquisitive and venturesome, who go places, do things, and explore new activities. People also make chance work for them by cultivating their interests, enabling beliefs and competencies. These personal resources enable them to make the most of opportunities that arise unexpectedly. Pasteur put it well when he noted, "Chance favors only the prepared mind." In a much earlier era, the philosopher Seneca portrayed seeming serendipity as "Luck is what happens when preparation meets opportunity." The harder one works, the luckier one gets. Even the distinguished lay philosopher Groucho Marx insightfully observed that people can influence how they play the hand fortuity deals them, "You have to be in the right place at the right time, but when it comes, you better have something on the ball." Personal development and engagement in a wide range of activities gives people a hand in shaping the courses their lives take.

AUTHOR NOTE

Some aspects of this entry include revised material from the following publications: Bandura, A. (2006). Toward a psychology of human agency. *Perspectives on Psychological Science, 1,* 164–180, and Bandura, A. (2005). The evolution of social cognitive theory. In K. G. Smith & M. A. Hitt (Eds.), *Great Minds in Management* (pp. 9–35). Oxford: Oxford University Press.

REFERENCES

Bandura, A. (1982). The psychology of chance encounters and life paths. *American Psychologist, 37,* 747–755.
Bandura, A. (1986). *Social foundations of thought and action: A social cognitive theory.* Englewood Cliffs, NJ: Prentice-Hall.
Bandura, A. (1998). Exploration of fortuitous determinants of life paths. *Psychological Inquiry, 9,* 95–99.
Bandura, A. (2002a). Growing primacy of human agency in adaptation and change in the electronic era. *European Psychologist, 7,* 2–16.
Bandura, A. (2002b). Social cognitive theory in cultural context. *Applied Psychology: An International Review, 51,* 269–90.

Bandura, A. (2006a). Toward a psychology of human agency. *Perspectives on Psychological Science, 1,* 164–80.

Bandura, A. (2006b). Going global with social cognitive theory: From prospect to paydirt. In S. I. Donaldson, D. E. Berger, & K. Pezdek (Eds.), *Applied psychology: New frontiers and rewarding careers* (pp. 53–79). Mahwah, NJ: Lawrence Erlbaum.

Bandura, A. (2008). The reconstrual of "free will" from the agentic perspective of social cognitive theory. In J. Baer, J. C. Kaufman & R. F. Baumeister (Eds.), *Are we free? Psychology and free will* (pp. 86–127). Oxford: Oxford University Press.

Harré, R., & Gillet, G. (1994). *The discursive mind.* Thousand Oaks, CA: Sage Publications.

Merton, R., & Barber, E. (2004). *The travels and adventures of serendipity.* Princeton: Princeton University Press.

PART II

Middle-Range Theories

JOHN DARLEY, Princeton University

Adventures in Rejectionland

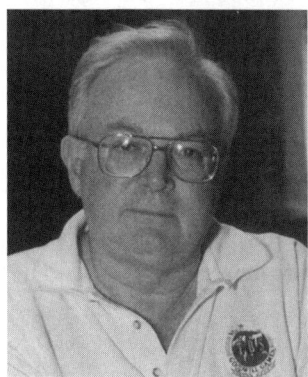

I was on a roll. My thesis, on fear and social comparison as determinants of conformity behavior, had claimed its rightful place in *JPSP*. (I somehow managed to overlook the extensive and generous manuscript editing by Bill McGuire, who my good luck had made the action editor on my thesis... Without going into embarrassing detail, I recall that the manuscript, as I sent it, had required more text pages for me to reveal all its glories than there were subjects in my sole thesis experiment.)

The two bystander papers that Bibb Latane and I did also found their way into *JPSP*. I *owned JPSP*!

So I decided to favor *JPSP* with another manuscript that contained another of my earth-shaking discoveries. And here the discovery was not just mine, but involved the contributions of Susan Darley and Tom Moriarty, among my best-ever graduate students, and Ellen Berscheid, a star from the Aronson Lab at Minnesota and a lifelong friend.

You can see where this is going. A rather terse rejection letter from *JPSP*—although not so terse that it missed the chance to cite the multiple reasons for the rejection. Devastated. I crept around the labs, head down. It took me weeks to convey its fate to my co-authors. Now that I look back at the publication date of the article that eventually found its way into print in *JESP*, I realize that it took me *years* to rewrite it for that submission.

There are lessons to be learned here, but before we get to them, I need to describe the rejected studies. What we should have said in the introduction of the article is this: "There is a remarkable contradiction in the ways in which sociologists, on the one hand, and psychologists, on the other, image two sets of conceptually similar actors. In sociology, it is the *deviants* who carry the stigma, in this case of deviance from social normality, the rest are *normal* citizens. In psychology, the *conformers* are the ones who carry the stigma of—in this instance—lack of moral courage to maintain independent attitudes and opinions, while it is the sturdy *independents*, in life and in Professor Asch's experiments, that we admire. But surely, there is some contradiction here. How is it that. . ." etc., etc.

We didn't begin the article with this framing, because I just had not asked myself what the core of the research was about, and made that the introduction to the experiment. A rookie mistake. Here is why I suspect I made it. I was inordinately proud of the clever twists we made on the Asch conformity study designs. In the now current vocabulary we had invented a *paradigm*. Blowing that methodological horn, I had not zeroed in on what Russ Fazio elsewhere in this book calls the "fundamental" contribution of the study.

The fundamental contribution is the contradiction that I pointed out above, and my colleagues and I demonstrated one aspect of it that could have contributed to the thinking that led to one of the major convergences of sociological and psychological social psychology. But my ponderous drafting style, my rookie inexperience with editor–author warfare, and my general timidity led first to a much-delayed publication that had lost any sense of what might be of interest in the article and any chance to give psychology an exciting new use of the Asch conformity paradigm.

Let me tell you about the study's central result. As we all know, in the Asch conformity paradigm, if there is one subject who is surrounded by the unanimous answers given by the others—others who seem to be normal subjects to the real subject but are confederates of the experimenter, giving unanimous prearranged wrong answers—then often the subject conforms. But if one of the confederates gives a correct response, the subject is freed to give the correct answer and almost always does so. This is the famous "minority of two condition." This result is true in the Asch original experiments, in which it is the length of lines that are judged, but also the case if it is the subject's opinions that are reported, as was demonstrated in subsequent experiments.

So in the minority of two condition the subject has given an answer uninfluenced by the majority, and we speak of him as "independent." But, if we stop to think, we realize that the subject has been independent with a little help from the co-reporting confederate. How should we conceptualize that help, and where might it lead the subject if we created opportunities in the experiment for it to lead somewhere interesting?

We don't know. The Asch experiment stopped here, as soon as the subject registered the "independent" answer. But it need not have stopped. So let us vary the experiment to create opportunities to see how the subject is bonded to the confederate who agrees. This turns out to be easy to do. One simply makes the initial Asch minority of two condition the beginning, the independent manipulation of the experiment. Next, after the subject has given her generally independent answer when under pressure from the majority, we then pair the subject off with the previously agreeing confederate, send the two of them off together, and see how the subject orients to the confederate.

This is what we did. Notice that this experiment is going to take a great deal of social psychological "trade-craft" to make it seem real to the subjects. But having trained with Elliot Aronson and Merrill Carlsmith, master experimentalists, I thought we could bring it off. Here is what the subject must believe—first that a substantial number of other subjects were actually present when they were all simulated by a tape recording that was made in advance; and second, that we did not know the subjects' actual answers to the opinion questions we would ask, when we actually did. How did we bring off this second trick? The subjects knew that they had in fact written down their opinions in advance, but had kept the only copy of the page on which their opinions were recorded. So we could not possibly know them.

We knew them. Magic stores sell rigged clipboards, with a sheet of carbon paper under the top writing surface. We retrieved the clipboard before beginning the experiment and fished out the carbon of their opinions. This made us innocently proud of our deception skills, although this faded a bit when we noticed that we could also discover the pattern of their opinions by unobtrusively glancing at their answer page while they filled it out.

More stagecraft. Not wishing to pay a large cast of confederates, we faked their presence with previously tape-recorded opinions. But different subjects had different opinions on the issues. How did we know what opinions to tape record in advance? We asked subjects to agree or disagree on each opinion. For each opinion, the two-channel tape recorder had on one track the appropriate pattern of answers to play to the subject who disagreed on that issue, and on the other track had the answers to play to the agreeing subject. The researcher could switch which of the two tracks the subject heard. This of course was hellishly complicated, and required great concentration and skills on the part of the assistant, but in those days, the research assistants were giants that walked the earth.

We then "drew lots" for further pairings of the subjects, and lo and behold, in the interesting experimental condition, the subject was paired with the fellow minority member. We now needed to figure out what we wanted to test for. The obvious answer was to see if the previous "sturdy independent" would be so independent if he was placed under conformity pressure from the person who previously had provided support to him when he faced the original disagreement from the majority. So we tested that. Next each of this pair of subjects was asked to register an opinion on some new set of topics and again, the confederate answered first. (More switch throwing.) But this time the confederate, who previously had agreed with the subject on issues, thus standing up to the majority and giving the subject support, often disagreed on these new issues.

Subjects in this situation conformed to the confederate a lot. They conformed more in this condition than in all the control conditions. (The original article gives the control conditions.) Other measures suggested why this was so. During the minority of two experience, the subjects had come to like and feel drawn to the confederate who gave them validation and support in the face of otherwise unanimous disagreement.

So one way of saying what the Asch results mean is this: Asch did not discover a set of people whose "independence" became apparent when another person provided social support for their opinions. Instead, he created the beginnings of a deviant group, who might begin to be more affected by their shared opinions and agenda and more able to deviate from the majority agenda.

I think that some interesting and important experimental social psychological research could trace out the possibilities here. Given our new understandings of social cognition and our new techniques for probing cognitive structures, a good deal of illumination of the cognitive, motivational and emotional basis of deviance might be found.

But what I mainly see is that I did not pursue these leads. Instead, I became so discouraged by the negative reception of our initial forays that I failed to follow this direction. I mention this because I have often heard others say similar things: "I just let that research line go and did other things instead." Arkin's challenge has allowed me and others to wander through a rarely explored corner of our intellectual biographies, that corner where we stored away what felt like dead ends—but things that just might be worth examining again.

REFERENCE

Darley, J. M., Moriarty, T., Darley, S., & Berscheid, E. (1974). Increased conformity to a fellow deviant as a function of prior deviation. *Journal of Experimental Social Psychology, 10,* 211–223.

GERALD L. CLORE, University of Virginia

Thrilling Thoughts: How Changing Your Mind Intensifies Your Emotions

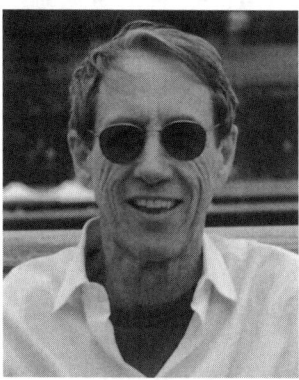

Imagine the experience of Captain El Tovar, who, in 1542, trudging through the wilderness of Arizona in search of the seven cities of gold, stumbled on the Grand Canyon. As he peered over the edge at the river 6000 feet below, how intense his experience of awe and amazement must have been!

And what of Oedipus, who, searching for the murderer of his father, King Laius, discovered that he himself was the guilty party, and that his wife Jocasta, therefore, was his own mother. These discoveries led her to hang herself and led Oedipus, with two pins from his dead mother's dress, to gouge out his eyes.

To contribute to the current volume, authors were asked to nominate something they had written that was underappreciated. My candidate is a brief essay (Clore, 1994), in which I asked what makes emotions intense. Part of my answer, as illustrated above, emphasized the role of experiencing cognitive structural change. Presumably, if we were to visit the Grand Canyon today, our experience would be less intense than that of the Spanish explorer, because we know a lot about it, have seen pictures, and may even have been there before. It would still be amazing, of course, but knowing what to expect should limit the amount of cognitive restructuring. In a related way, when vacationing in the mountains or on the ocean, it can be distressing how quickly one adapts to the surrounding beauty. Looking at photographs or thinking about the experience later can regenerate only some of the initial intensity. And as images lose their power to restructure our mental experience, the most we can hope for is a memory of the fact that we were once amazed.

After having one's world turned upside down, as happened to Oedipus, adaptation would be much more difficult. His trauma was fictional, but people do sometimes experience extreme cognitive restructuring. One might discover that one's spouse has been leading a double life or that one's parish priest is a child molester. Some people discover that their mother and father are not actually their birth parents, and in psychotherapy, people sometimes come to see themselves and their families in a new light that changes everything. In addition, sooner or later we all experience the death of someone close. When that happens, our mental representations of our lives may become dramatically restructured. I propose that just as the amount and rate that one descends on a roller coaster determines the intensity of that experience, the amount and rate of change in cognitive structure may determine the intensity of emotional experiences.

EMOTIONAL INTENSITY

Some of the more specific factors that make emotions intense or mild differ for different emotions (Ortony, Clore, & Collins, 1988). For example, fear is more intense when a feared outcome is especially important. Thus, fearing for one's life should be more intense than fearing that one will be late for work. Fear is also more intense when the feared outcome seems more rather than less likely to occur. By contrast, the intensity of the emotion of shame depends not on the likelihood of bad outcomes, but on the blameworthiness of one's actions. Shame is more intense if one violates an especially important standard or feels especially responsible. But underlying even these specific and local factors, I suggest, is the role of cognitive restructuring, a more general phenomenological factor that I see as the ultimate, the real, intensity variable.

If this idea seems unfamiliar, that may reflect the lack of attention it attracted 15 years ago when it was first published. Whereas people on the street know what "cognitive dissonance" is, "cognitive restructuring" is relatively unknown even in psychology. But of course, dissonance was elaborated by its author in many publications over many years, whereas restructuring was mentioned only once in a short chapter in a long book.

But I am still quite attracted to this restructuring hypothesis. It handles nicely the fact that satisfying pieces of humor, music, and literature, for example, all require a sufficiently well-developed cognitive structure for one to be moved. Thus, classical and jazz pieces are most satisfying when an initial theme is sufficiently accessible that one can take delight in its rhythmic and melodic transformation. And the endings of Dickens' novels are especially pleasing because there are lots of structural changes as the characters' lives suddenly intersect, and all is resolved.

A primary source of appreciation of novels, plays, and films lies in readers' and viewers' perceptions of the ways in which characters develop and change as events unfold. A fascinating variation on this requirement can be seen in the 1984 German film *Sugar Baby*, which shows the development of a romance between a fat woman who is a mortician and a much younger subway conductor. In this understated film, the most important changes are in viewers' feelings about the characters rather than in the characters themselves. Viewers find at some point that their initial feelings of discomfort and repulsion have changed. Instead of seeing only the mortician's unappealing fatness and other incongruities, one finds oneself disarmed by the universal beauty of the romance between these two otherwise lonely people. In terms of our hypothesis, *Sugar Baby* is satisfying because of the change we experience in ourselves and what we care about. And the more dramatically we experience such change, the more satisfying we should find the film.

Note, however, that such cognitive structural change is not the same as raw stimulus change. If scenes from one film or book or piece of music were simply stuck into the middle of another work, there might be much stimulus change, but little change in one's cognitive model of what went before. On the other hand, recent research shows that although people prefer their television programs to be uninterrupted, commercial interruptions actually increase enjoyment by disrupting the process of adaptation (Nelson, Meyvis, & Galak, 2009). Thus, although such interruptions do not change the story, they do require that one transport oneself back and forth between the fictional world being depicted and one's everyday world. These results suggest that the critical variable lies in the *experience* of structural change, not in the structural change itself.

RELATED IDEAS

Writers focusing on related ideas include Keltner and Haidt's (2003) proposals about the emotion of awe. They propose that awe involves both perceptions of vastness and a need for accommodation. A charismatic leader, a grand vista, and a symphony might all elicit awe. They maintain that experiences that lack one or both of these features do not qualify as awe. Thus, for example, they say that "surprise" involves accommodation without vastness.

Some empirical research also focuses on ideas related to our hypothesis. For example, long-time colleague Bob Wyer proposed a wonderful theory of humor (Wyer & Collins, 1992) in which the critical factor is an experience of some kind of diminishment. The diminishment can take many forms. In the classic form of cartoons and jokes, high-status individuals might be brought low by a banana peel, or people representing racial, ethnic, or gender stereotypes might get diminished in various ways. In addition, listeners to jokes invariably experience a kind of diminishment when the arrival of the punch line makes it clear that they were pursuing the wrong assumptions about where the joke was going. But the change is nevertheless experienced by most people as enjoyable, and presumably more cognitive restructuring results in more appreciation and laughter. But in addition to the amount, the rate of cognitive change is also critical, since in humor, timing is everything.

If these principles predict how funny people find humor, might they also predict how people experience insights as profound? If humor involves cognitive change in the direction of some kind of diminishment, perhaps the experience of profundity involves cognitive changes in the direction of some kind of elevation or expansion of ideas. If a saying or analogy in which a topic is diminished is funny (e.g., "Lectures are like sleeping pills"), perhaps an analogy in which a topic gets elevated seems profound (e.g., "Libraries are like gold mines"). In any event, the size of the change experienced as one comprehends the humor or insight should be related to the degree of satisfaction.

The single most elegant study of the process we have in mind is not well known, because it is described only in a book chapter on metaphor (Sternberg, Tourangeau, & Nigro, 1979). It involved the creation of metaphors based on the multidimensional scaling of various domains in order to establish psychological distances among the elements. Consistent with our hypothesis, the most satisfying metaphors had specific elements that were very similar, but that were in domains that were very different from each other. That is, as long as the elements fit, the greater the mental travel or cognitive remapping involved, the more people were likely to smile and say, "Ahh, what a satisfying metaphor!"

In related work, Dougal and Schooler (2007) studied the effects of having an "ah-ha" experience as one solves anagrams. In unpublished research, Schooler had participants solve anagrams before they got the punch lines of jokes. He found that the "ah-ha" experience of solving an anagram was sufficiently similar to the "ah-ha" experience of understanding the punch line that anagram solving made jokes funnier. Again, the intensity of affect depended on the total amount of cognitive restructuring experienced.

When I related this idea to Kay Deaux recently, she countered by saying that some narratives are riveting even when one knows how the story ends and there is no surprise or restructuring involved. That is an excellent point. But when novels or films start with a defining event, so that the rest consists of flashbacks, knowing the end point may even increase the number of mental trips that readers or viewers implicitly make back and forth. If so, then the sum of the experiences of cognitive change may get multiplied. Suspense may intensify one's experience in a related way, because one implicitly entertains first one outcome and then the opposite. Such flip-flopping of one's cognitive model involves lots of restructuring experiences and hence lots of potential for emotional intensity. Again, apparently the critical variable is not the restructuring itself, but the associated experience.

Before closing, I should mention that the current phenomenological hypothesis is intended to be more broadly applicable than has so far been discussed. For example, I believe that other emotion intensity variables, such as goal importance, reduce to the same thing. The relative importance of various goals, values, or attitudes is often quite difficult to specify. But within the current hypothesis, their importance would simply be the extent that they are central within their respective structures. Goal importance, then, would be the degree to which a unit of change in a given goal alters other goals and plans to which it is linked. For example, the well-being of one's spouse is usually quite a central goal, and the death of a spouse affects many other aspects of a person's life. To the extent that it does, it would clearly be an important goal, and having that goal thwarted should be met with intense and enduring emotional reactions reflecting the amount and rate of cognitive structural change that is experienced.

AUTHOR NOTE

Support is acknowledged from National Institute of Mental Health Research Grant MH50074.

REFERENCES

Clore, G. L. (1994). Why emotions vary in intensity. In P. Ekman & R. J. Davidson (Eds.), *The nature of emotion: Fundamental questions* (pp. 386–393). New York: Oxford University Press.

Dougal, S., & Schooler, J. W. (2007). Discovery misattribution: When solving is confused with remembering. *Journal of Experimental Psychology: General, 136,* 577–592.

Keltner, D., & Haidt, J. (2003). Approaching awe: A moral, spiritual, and aesthetic emotion. *Cognition & Emotion, 17,* 297–314.

Nelson, L. D., Meyvis, T., & Galak, J. (2009). Enhancing the television-viewing experience through commercial interruptions. *Journal of Consumer Research, 36* 160–172.

Ortony, A., Clore, G. L., & Collins, A. (1988). *The cognitive structure of emotions.* New York: Cambridge University Press.

Sternberg, R. J., Tourangeau, R., & Nigro, G. (1979). Metaphor, induction, and social policy: The convergence of macroscopic and microscopic views. In A. Ortony (Ed.), *Metaphor and thought* (pp. 325–353). New York: Cambridge University Press.

Wyer, R. S., & Collins, J. (1992). The theory of humor elicitation. *Psychological Review, 99,* 663–688.

RUSSELL H. FAZIO, Ohio State University

A Fundamental Conceptual
Distinction . . . Gone Unnoticed

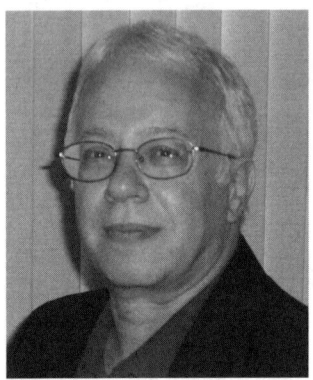

I do not believe that I have ever prepared a manuscript without a strong sense of enthusiasm regarding the importance of the work and the contribution it offered. Indeed, the eager anticipation of the impact that I am convinced a paper-in-preparation will have regularly facilitates its reaching fruition. In some instances, that anticipation has been justified. The work has been read and cited, and hind-sight shows it to have nudged the field's thinking in the direction I had envisioned. On occasion, a work's impact has far exceeded even the wildest expectations I could have ever imagined. However, the opposite has also been true. What I viewed at the time (and in a few cases continue to view to this day) as a brilliant conceptual insight or remarkable empirical finding has languished in the literature, largely unnoticed by the scientific community.

One of the languished has been especially striking, even poignant to me, for a long time now. Hence, when my colleague and friend Bob Arkin, in his role as editor of this volume, posed the challenge of identifying my "most underappreciated" work, little or no latency was involved. (A good deal of my more appreciated work speaks to the telling nature of responses offered with quick latency, so I place considerable trust in my effortless reaction.) The answer clearly had to be my dissertation work.

In all likelihood, the poignancy to which I referred stems from this having been my dissertation. When introducing a class to a significant piece of research, I have always taken considerable delight in identifying it as some now eminent scientist's dissertation. Somehow, that little tidbit of trivia seems to personalize the science and, at the same time, illustrate its cumulative nature. The passing comment connotes that even very recognized scholars were once students earnestly committed to the completion of a PhD thesis. I am quite sure my own dissertation has never been featured in this way (other than the lecture equivalent of a self-citation, that is). Indeed, I suspect that only a very small number of people, few beyond my advisor and my spouse, could even identify what I did as my dissertation research. Although published in the *Journal of Personality and Social Psychology* (Fazio, 1979), the article reporting this research never garnered much attention: As of 2010, it had averaged all of 1.19 citations per year.

Yet, I continue to look back at the work with considerable pride, as well as with the counterfactual musings of what might have been. Its essence concerned what I termed the "construction–validation distinction"—collecting information about an object for the purpose of constructing a judgment of it, versus testing the validity of a judgment already reached. The distinction centered on the nature of information being sought, information about the object versus information about one's judgment of the object. I described the construction motive as parallel to a researcher's conducting an exploratory investigation with the intent of gathering data that would facilitate the generation of hypotheses, whereas the validation motive was akin to conducting an empirical test of a hypothesis.

The distinction was prompted by, and embedded within, social comparison theory. At the time, Festinger's theory was enjoying a resurgence of interest, evidenced by the publication of Suls and Miller's influential edited volume reviewing theoretical and empirical perspectives on social comparison processes. Among those developments was the one that most influenced my own thinking—the attributional perspective espoused by Al Goethals and John Darley (1977). With the benefit of invaluable input from my advisor Joel Cooper, the dissertation project linked the construction–validation distinction to the longstanding issue in the social comparison literature regarding choice of comparison other. Drawing upon Goethals and Darley's analysis of the value of triangulating evidence and the characteristics of a comparison other most likely to provide such triangulation, I argued that a validation motive would be best served by someone who showed evidence of agreeing with one's judgment despite their being rather dissimilar on dimensions related to the judgment. As Goethals and Darley had noted, agreement from dissimilar others, by virtue of the different perspective they bring to bear on the judgment, provides evidence that one's own judgment emanates from the entity in question and not some personal idiosyncrasy. In contrast, a construction motive, I argued, might be best served by engagement with a similar disagreer. The commonality in terms of relevant attributes suggests that such a person should be agreeing with one's own judgment. The disagreement implies that the person may possess some information about the entity that you yourself lack.

This reasoning was supported in a series of three experiments, ones for which I fondly remember the process of data collection. Indeed, these had to rank among the occasions in which I most enjoyed the experimenter role. The procedure involved the elaborate staging of a ruse to convince participants of the presence of co-participants, which required such foolishness as stomping loudly along the corridor in heavy boots, repeatedly opening and closing the doors to empty booths, and talking to nonexistent people. Moreover, the experiments, which purportedly concerned "the perceptual judgment of motion and distance," focused on the autokinetic effect as the judgments of interest. As Sherif had demonstrated decades earlier, estimating the distance that a dot of light appears to move in a completely dark room is fraught with ambiguity. Presumably to simulate different ways in which judgments are made, participants undertook a series of trials in which they offered independent judgments, followed by a series in which they were informed of each other's judgments at the end of each trial (during which agreement was manipulated). This was to be followed by a "coalition series" during which pairs of participants would discuss their judgments over an intercom system prior to reaching a joint decision. Partner selection was the major dependent measure.

Some of the experiments also involved the manipulation of similarity or dissimilarity with respect to "perceptual style." This was accomplished via the provision of bogus test profiles on what were purported to be perceptual tests of depth versus lateral perception. To foster concerns with construction versus validation, participants' perceived level of information about the distance that the light might move was manipulated. Participants were led to believe that they would be assigned to one of three conditions involving varying degrees of information about the light's likely movement: range information for each trial, range information for the trials as a whole, or no information at all. They then found themselves assigned to one of these latter two conditions, thus being relatively advantaged or disadvantaged compared to some others in the group. This factor influenced participants' preferences for a partner. Those who had been led to believe that they were somewhat advantaged informationally found the "dissimilar agreer" more attractive than those who had been disadvantaged, presumably because this partner satisfied a desire for validation. In contrast, those with no information preferred the "similar disagreer" to a greater extent than those who had been provided with partial information, presumably because this partner was likely to possess useful information about the light's movement.

I certainly thought the findings were exciting and, hence, I expected the article to have more impact than it did. Why did it fall flat? A number of factors may have played a role. In hindsight, the surge of interest in social comparison processes appears to have been brief, already having passed its peak by the time the article was published. Moreover, I now recognize how unusual it is for any solitary article to produce a substantial impact. Typically, any well-cited article generates attention because of its featured role in a broader program of research. Significant advances tend be achieved by research programs, not by one-shot articles. And, therein lay those counterfactual musings. What if I had pursued that line of research? At the time, I was heavily engaged in a research program on attitude–behavior consistency and the conditions, especially the attitudinal qualities, that promoted such consistency. Indeed, this work predated my interest in social comparison processes, and I had a good sense of the future direction it needed to take. It was one of those lines of work for which the next study to be done, the next question to be asked, the next hypothesis to be tested, consistently seemed to emerge naturally from the previous findings. That was one of the reasons I found it so engaging. In contrast, I seemed incapable of identifying the next step in the social comparison work.

Here the counterfactuals grow all the stronger for me. What if I had been smart enough to recognize the real promise of the dissertation research? With the benefit of hindsight, I now realize that I could not discern where to take the social comparison research precisely because I had categorized it as social comparison work. That seemed to blind me to its true value. There was an aspect of the work far more fundamental than any questions regarding choice of comparison other, and that was the very distinction between construction and validation. These are not just "motives for social comparison," as I had entitled the dissertation and the *JPSP* article, but much more general motivations relevant to judgmental processes. Construction and validation are central to issues of information acquisition, hypothesis generation, hypothesis testing, the conclusion that one has arrived at a sufficiently valid judgment, and the confidence one places in that judgment. At its heart, the construction–validation distinction highlights the importance of the point in a judgmental sequence at which individuals feel that they have enough information about a question to begin to entertain specific answers—that is, the point at which they are sufficiently satisfied with the information they have acquired to begin to test hypotheses. It is at this point that the focus of information acquisition shifts from the object to the judgment of the object. Moreover, there is a dynamic interplay between the two motivational goals. Satisfactory construction promotes the desire for validation, and failures to validate are likely to prompt a return to a construction state and a search for additional relevant information. Given all that the field has come to know about the confirmation biases that often accompany hypothesis testing, the shift from construction to validation also represents the onset of a less open-minded perspective regarding the issue.

Over the years, as I witnessed the advances in our knowledge regarding such matters as hypothesis testing, meta-cognition, confidence, and openness to new information, I frequently thought of the distinction between construction and validation. As a result, I now see the conceptual framework as much more central than I had envisioned earlier, and certainly as extending far beyond the consideration of social comparison processes. So, if any lesson were to be gleaned from what I personally wish to regard as a "hidden gem," it might be the value of focusing on *the fundamental* —that is, the aspect of the conceptual reasoning with the broadest and most far-reaching implications. What may be most likely to offer a significant, long-term contribution and, hence, what may most merit the investment of time and effort, is the question, the level of analysis, or the finding that is the more fundamental. That consideration should carry substantial weight when making decisions about the potential directions a research program might take: Always look toward the more fundamental.

REFERENCES

Fazio, R. H. (1979). Motives for social comparison: The construction-validation distinction. *Journal of Personality and Social Psychology, 37,* 1683–1698.

Goethals, G. R., & Darley, J. M. (1977). Social comparison theory: An attributional approach. In J. M. Suls & R. L. Miller (Eds.), *Social comparison processes: Theoretical and empirical perspectives* (pp. 259–278). Washington, DC: Hemisphere.

MARGARET S. CLARK, Yale University

Communal Relationships Can Be Selfish and Give Rise to Exploitation

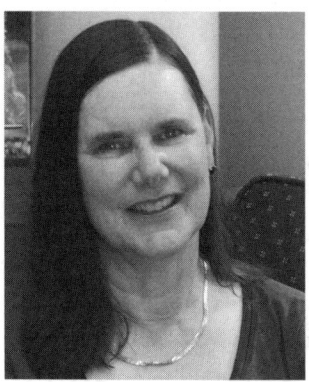

My work with Judson Mills on the distinction between communal and exchange relationships has been around for over 30 years. Much of it is well cited. I'm pleased. Yet the claims made in the title of this piece still comes as a surprise to many people. Indeed, our original qualitative distinction often has been interpreted as one between cold, *selfish* exchange relationships and lovely, warm and fuzzy, *unselfish* communal ones. It's not. We've said so in many theoretical pieces. We've said that desire for mutual communal relationships normatively should lead you to focus on what partners are doing *for you* and have empirically demonstrated that it does (Clark, Dubash, & Mills, 1998). We have outlined how adoption of a communal norm sets the stage for distinctive types of exploitation that are violations of communal norms but arise in these relationships (Mills & Clark, 1986). Almost no one cites these papers.[1] The sometimes selfish side of communal relationships is never mentioned in texts (nor is the sometimes selfless side of exchange relationships).

THE DISTINCTION IS NOT ONE OF SELFISH VERSUS UNSELFISH RELATIONSHIPS

The original, qualitative, distinction and follow-ups emphasizing variation in communal strength have to do with the norms governing the giving and receipt of benefit (see Clark & Mills, 2011). In exchange relationships benefits are given with the expectation of receiving a comparable benefit in return (or in response to benefits received in the past.) In communal relationships benefits are given, non-contingently, to promote the welfare of the partner. These points are made accurately in texts, and it's easy to see why the former norm seems selfish (one gives to get something) and the latter selfless (one gives to promote another's welfare). But there's more to the story.

First, one must consider motives for adopting each of these norms in the first place. Motives for adopting and implementing a communal norm can be relatively selfless *or selfish*. Motives for adopting and implementing an exchange norm can be relatively selfish *or selfless*.

Consider adopting a communal norm first. *After* a communal norm is adopted, benefits are given non-contingently, *but* either selfish or unselfish motives can drive a person to adopt the norm in the first place. If I have just moved to a new community, wish to form new friendships, and act on a communal basis toward potential friends with the goal of starting a friendship, I have adopted a communal norm for selfish reasons. If I care for a disagreeable, elderly relative on a communal basis to avoid guilt or criticism from other people, I have adopted a communal norm for selfish reasons. Despite my initial selfish motives, however, the norm, once adopted, then leads me to non-contingently provide support to others to advance their welfare. There also exist unselfish reasons for following a communal norm. Empathy is one. People often do feel empathy in response to another's distress, adopt a communal norm, and then act non-contingently, with their primary goal being to alleviate another's suffering—a process that likely drives much charitable giving.[2] There are likely other motives, even hard-wired motives, automatic, unconscious, ones such as the drive to care for one's offspring that lead to adherence to a communal norm that would at least appear unselfish. Some, of course, say that they are selfish in the sense of promoting the survival of one's genes across generations. Honestly, though, whereas we recognize the existence of interesting debates regarding whether truly selfless acts exist, that question is not the basis for our work.

Next consider motives for adopting an exchange norm, which also may be relatively selfish or selfless. The selfish ones are easy to point out. If I go to the store to buy a loaf of bread, it is for selfish reasons. I want that bread. I'm not thinking of the grocer's welfare. When I formed a carpool to drive my daughter to a pool for swim practice, I wasn't terribly concerned with helping out other parents, nor was it likely they opted in thinking of my welfare: We all wanted to save time and drive less. Yet there can be mixed selfish and unselfish motives or even mostly unselfish reasons for adopting an exchange norm as well. I might buy fair trade coffee (instead of equally good and less expensive coffee) because I think coffee growers should get a fair exchange for their product. I might hire an unemployed person to help with a task in bad economic times (even when I could do the task easily and less expensively myself) because I think it is the right thing to do.

In discussing whether communal relationships are selfish or not, it is important to make two additional points. First, many (not all) communal relationships are mutual or symmetrical ones. People in these relationships not only expect to be non-contingently responsive to partners' needs and desires as appropriate; they also expect their partners to be non-contingently responsive to their own welfare. The balance of the actual benefits does not have to be even; but in mutual, symmetrical communal relationships, concern for one another's welfare is expected to be even at least so long as both members retain the ability to be equally responsive to the other. Long ago Utne, Hatfield, Traupman, and Greenberger (1984) published an article in which they argued that equity theory applied to intimate relationships. They cited us as skeptics who claimed that "intimate relationships are 'special'—the reciprocity rules that apply in almost all other encounters are said to be left at the door when one enters a truly intimate relationship" (p. 325). I think they meant we were overly romantic in conceptualizing communal relationships as unselfish and thought us naïve. Yet, in fact, we were not arguing that reciprocity (generally conceptualized) is irrelevant to communal relationships. In mutual, symmetric communal relationships (e.g., friendships, many romantic relationships) people do expect a distinctly communal type of reciprocity. It is reciprocity of concerns for needs and responsiveness to needs and desires *as they arise*. Each benefit is still given non-contingently; needs (and thus benefit provision) can be unequal if needs are unequal and record-keeping of actual inputs into the relationships is inappropriate (although violations of norms do occur). Moreover, you really can't demand that another attend to your needs if they fail to do so, nor can you take them to court. Yet in mutual communal relationships tracking whether the other is responsive to your needs is appropriate and does occur (see the neglected Clark, Dubash, & Mills, 1998, piece). If needs are neglected one may express hurt (a uniquely communal word) and hope the other feels guilt and responds. Alternatively, one can choose to leave the relationship; one need not be an unselfish martyr. What one can't do (while still adhering to a communal norm) is to demand repayment of concern.[3] The term "reciprocity" is imprecise. Researchers need to specify exactly what it means to them. We assert it means something distinct in communal as compared to exchange relationships.

Second, people have hierarchies of communal relationships (and assume more communal responsibility for those higher in their hierarchies). This fact relates to the quantitative dimension of communal relationships (another oft-neglected point we have made). Importantly, they place *themselves* in their own hierarchies, typically high in those hierarchies. It means that most people do consider taking care of their own needs to take precedence over taking care of most other people's needs, even when it may be said that they have communal relationships with those others. It is easy to illustrate this. People send themselves, not their neighbors or friends, on vacation (but they still can act communally toward those friends within the cost boundaries dictated by the communal strength of their relationship with that person).

THE NEGLECTED PAPERS

Our two neglected papers focus on people's self-interest in relationships. In one we report three studies showing that, when led to desire a communal relationship, people are especially likely to track whether a partner is demonstrating concern for their own needs. They are especially likely to attend to how much time someone spends selecting hints to give them on a task they must perform (Clark, Dubash, & Mills, 1998, Studies 1 & 2) and in how much time partners report they would spend to select a gift for them, whether partners would give the same gift to another person, and how much the gift cost (Clark et al., 1998, Study 3). Moreover, they are even more motivated to do so when they are uncertain about the others' care for them (Clark et al., 1998, Studies 2 & 3). Our other neglected paper is a theoretical one in which we discuss the different ways in which people may exploit one another after adopting a communal versus an exchange norm (Mills & Clark, 1986). Whereas exaggerating the value of something one gave to another may be a good technique for exploitation in an exchange relationship (because it suggests they owe you more in return), it isn't a great exploitative technique in a communal relationships (where, instead, it suggests how much you care). Different exploitative techniques appear in communal relationships. Exaggerating one's own needs (thereby suggesting the other should do more for you than you truly need) and minimizing their needs (suggesting one need do less for them) are exploitative techniques common to communal and not exchange relationship. They may be infrequently studied by relationship researchers but are well known by all social beings involved in close relationships and are captured in lay language (e.g., the term "guilt trip").

ARE WE TO BLAME FOR THE NEGLECT OF THESE TWO ARTICLES?

I suspect there are two reasons these two papers have been neglected (in addition to the one paper having been left off electronic databases). One is not our fault. It is simply that the question of whether behavior is ever unselfish or is it purely selfish *is* a very interesting philosophical and psychological question that has captured the interest of many people. It's not our central question, but I believe it has been projected onto our work by others.

However, we are partially responsible. In selecting dependent variables on which to focus we've chosen ones that *seem* (on the surface, if one doesn't consider the theoretical points made above) intrinsically unselfish. We have shown that when people have or desire communal relationships (relative to those who have or desire exchange relationships), they like partners who do not pay them back for favors more than those who do, do not keep track of individual inputs into joint tasks but do track partner needs, help partners more, like and are more responsive to partners' emotional expressions, and feel especially good after helping their partners and especially bad after refusing to help their partners, all relative to what occurs in exchange relationships (see Clark & Mills, 2011, for a review). We have only rarely selected ones (e.g., keeping track of a partner's concern for the self, exaggerating needs) that are seemingly selfish.

In closing, I express my gratitude to Judson Mills for forcing me to be clear regarding my own thinking about the issues discussed here and for clearly being the one of the two of us who emphasized the importance of our conducting the Clark et al. (1998) research and writing the Mills and Clark (1986) paper. I believe he would be pleased to see the work defended here. I know this piece would be more precise and concisely written had he joined me in writing it.

NOTES

1. In preparing this piece I attempted to access the Clark et al, 1998 article using PsycARTI-CLES as well as using PsycINFO and was surprised to note that this *Journal of Experimental Social Psychology* paper appears in neither data base. This likely has contributed to the neglect. At my request this paper now has been added to the PsychARTICLES data base.
2. It is also worth noting that adopting a communal norm, then focusing on another's welfare itself almost certainly increases empathy (see Batson, Eklund, Hakansson, Chermok, Hoyt & Ortiz, 2007) resulting in enhanced responsiveness to partners. If the original motive to adopt the norm is selfish but then adopting the norm increases empathically based responsiveness, is the responsiveness selfish or unselfishly motivated. I'd say it is both.
3. I hasten to add that asymmetrical communal relationships without much expected reciprocity of attention to needs also exist—for example, the relationships many concerned and devoted parents have with their disabled children.

REFERENCES

Batson, C. D., Hakansson, J., Chermok, V.L., Hoyt, J.L., & Ortiz, B.G. (2007). An additional antecedent of empathic concern: Valuing the welfare of the person in need. *Journal of Personality and Social Psychology, 93*, 65–74.

Clark, M. S., & Mills, J. (in press, 2011). A theory of communal (and exchange) relationships. In P. A. M. Van Lange, A. W. Kruglanski, & E. T. Higgins (Eds.), *Handbook of theories of social psychology*. Thousand Oaks, CA: Sage Publications, Inc.

Clark, M. S., Dubash, P., & Mills, J. (1998). Interest in another's consideration of one's needs. *Journal of Experimental Social Psychology, 34*, 246–264.

Mills, J., & Clark, M. S. (1986). Communications that should lead to perceived exploitation in communal and exchange relationships. *Journal of Social and Clinical Psychology, 4*, 225–234.

Utne, M. K., Hatfield, E., Traupmann, J., & Greenberger, D. (1984). Equity, marital satisfaction, and stability. *Journal of Social and Personal Relationships, 3*, 323–332.

TIMOTHY D. WILSON, University of Virginia

Take Me Out to the Ballgame

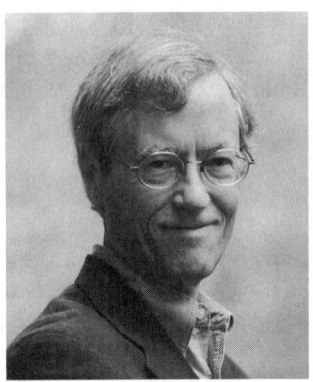

Imagine you arrive at a movie theater with high hopes—your friends have been raving about the latest Julia Roberts feature and you have been looking forward to seeing it all week. You settle into your seat, with a delicious-smelling tub of popcorn in your lap, eager for the lights to dim and the coming attractions to end. But suppose the movie isn't all that it's cracked up to be. In fact, it's a mundane, forgettable film that won't make anyone's list of best movies. How, if at all, will your high expectations influence your actual enjoyment of the film?

Some of my graduate students and I decided to investigate this question more than 20 years ago. To our surprise there was little research on how people's affective expectations influenced their affective experiences. There was research on the effects of expectations about the occurrence of an event (e.g., how likely I believe it is that my friends will throw me a surprise party), but no one had looked at the effects of expectations about one's affective reactions (how enjoyable I think such a party will be).

One reason this question had been neglected, perhaps, is that the answer seemed obvious. We can all think of times when we were disappointed because something did not live up to our expectations. If we expect to love a movie, and it is mediocre, we are disappointed and will probably like the movie less than if we had had no expectations. This would be an example of an affective contrast effect.

It seemed to us, however, that an assimilation effect might occur instead, especially if expectations lead to theory-driven processing of the event. If we are perched at the edge of our seat, ready to be wowed by a first-rate film, maybe we won't notice that the plot is overcomplicated and that our favorite actor is not turning in her best performance. There is plenty of evidence for confirmation biases in the realm of judgment; why should affective experience be any less theory-driven?

We conducted a series of studies that addressed these questions and reported them in two empirical papers (Wilson, Lisle, Kraft, & Wetzel, 1989; Klaaren, Hodges, & Wilson, 1994) and one review chapter (Wilson & Klaaren, 1992). We found that affective expectations *did* influence how people processed an event and their enjoyment of it, with assimilation effects being much more common than contrast effects. In one study, for example, people who expected a series of cartoons to be funny rated them as funnier and laughed at them more than people who had no expectations. In addition, they spent significantly less time looking at the cartoons, presumably because they did a quick "confirmation check," failed to notice that the cartoons were inconsistent with their expectations, and saw no need to process them further (Wilson et al., 1989). In other words, affective expectations led to top-down assimilation, not contrast.

This led to another question that (to me, at least) seemed even more interesting: What happens over time when people recognize that their affective expectations were disconfirmed? Will a decision whether to repeat the experience be guided by one's original expectations or the memory of what it was really like? We suspected the former, based in part on an experience of mine, in which I, an avid baseball fan, drove 70 miles to take my young kids to a minor league baseball game. What could be more fun than taking the family to America's favorite pastime, I figured, where we could enjoy well-played games while eating hotdogs and munching on peanuts? Well, anyone who has taken young children to sporting events knows the answer. A three-year-old couldn't care less what was happening on the diamond; what on earth are those men doing wearing strange outfits and carrying sticks and big gloves, anyway? My kids, at least, found it much more interesting to play in the gravel under the stands, where I had to keep them from kicking up dust and bothering the other spectators. Then there was the long drive home after the game, when everyone was tired and cranky. At the end of the trip I vowed never to go back, at least not until my kids were old enough to prefer the game to the gravel.

But by the time the next summer rolled around, my original expectations were more powerful than my memory for the actual experience the year before. How bad could it have been? It's America's favorite pastime! Sure, I spent a lot of time under the stands in the gravel last year, but I got to watch some of the game, and besides, my son is four now! Off we went, and it was only on the long drive home that I (once again) realized that my expectations were no match for reality.

We bottled this experience in a lab study in which we manipulated two things independently: people's expectations about an affective experience and the quality of the experience itself (Klaaren et al., 1994). In brief, participants watched a Charlie Chaplin film in the lab, with half the participants first being told that prior participants had loved it (which raised their expectations). Crossed with that manipulation, half watched the film under comfortable conditions and half under unpleasant conditions (they had to place their chins on an uncomfortable chin rest and watch a blurry copy of the film at a 45-degree angle). Both manipulations influenced people's enjoyment of the film: People liked it more if they expected to like it and they liked it more if they saw it under normal than degraded viewing conditions. We then telephoned people a few weeks later and asked them if they wanted to come back and watch another Charlie Chaplin film under the exact same viewing conditions as they had watched the first film. As we predicted, only people's expectations influenced their decision about whether to come back. People who had originally expected to enjoy the film were more willing to return, even if they had watched the film under unpleasant conditions. It was like my baseball game experience—after some time had passed, people's expectations trumped their memories of the experience itself.

This seemed like a pretty cool finding to us, one that had lots of implications for affective experiences in everyday life. But while the reaction to this work was not exactly resounding silence, neither was it overwhelming. The 1989 paper, published in the *Journal of Personality and Social Psychology*, has been cited 85 times—nothing to sneeze at, but still less than we expected. The 1994 paper, published in *Social Cognition*, has been cited 54 times, and the review chapter has been cited only 38 times. Perhaps even more telling is that other researchers, with a couple of exceptions, have not followed up on this work.

What lessons are to be learned from this? It is important, obviously, to choose research topics that seem important and resonate with one's personal experiences, rather than relying only on whatt other people think is important. Some of the best work in social psychology has been inspired by researchers' observations of their own lives, not from reading the journals. At the same time, there can be wisdom in crowds, and if one's findings continue to fall flat with multiple audiences, that is informative. In fact, I have a confession to make: In preparing this piece I went back and reread the 1994 article that reported the "Charlie Chaplin" study and my reaction was . . . well . . . it *was* a cool study, but the results weren't nearly as clean and airtight as I had remembered. I seem to have had an overly positive memory of this study, perhaps stemming from my initial enthusiasm and expectations for it—just as the theory predicts!

Undoubtedly there are other reasons why these studies didn't get the attention we thought they deserved. Other researchers did a much better job than we did of demonstrating exactly when assimilation versus contrast effects occur in the affective realm (Geers & Lassiter, 1999, 2002). The studies did not fit neatly into existing research areas, such as attitudes, social cognition, or emotion. Perhaps most tellingly, it was not obvious, to us anyway, what the next big question was in this area, and so our attention turned to other topics. But, in the end I did learn one thing from all of this—to wait until my kids were a lot older before taking them to another baseball game.

REFERENCES

Geers, A., & Lassiter, G. (1999). Affective expectations and information gain: Evidence for assimilation and contrast effects in affective experience. *Journal of Experimental Social Psychology, 35*, 394–413.

Geers, A., & Lassiter, G. (2002). Effects of affective expectations on affective experience: The moderating role of optimism-pessimism. *Personality and Social Psychology Bulletin, 28*, 1026–1039.

Klaaren, K. J., Hodges, S. D., & Wilson, T. D. (1994). The role of affective expectations in subjective experience and decision making. *Social Cognition, 12*, 77–101.

Wilson, T. D., & Klaaren, K. (1992). The role of affective expectations in affective experience. In M. S. Clark (Ed.), *Review of personality and social psychology: Emotion and social behavior* (Vol. 14, pp. 1–31). Newbury Park, CA: Sage.

Wilson, T. D., Lisle, D. J., Kraft, D., & Wetzel, C. G. (1989). Preferences as expectation-driven inferences: Effects of affective expectations on affective experience. *Journal of Personality and Social Psychology, 56*, 519–30.

MILES HEWSTONE, University of Oxford, UK

Timing Is Everything . . . At Least for Citation Impact

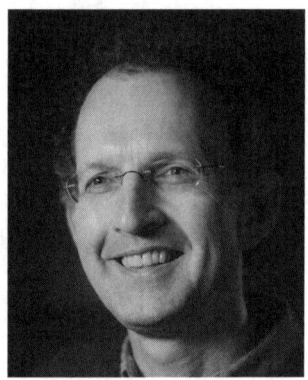

"There is only one thing in the world worse than being talked about, and that is not being talked about." Oscar Wilde, *The Picture of Dorian Gray* (1891)
"For everything there is a season, and a time for every matter under heaven."
(Ecclesiastes, 3:1–15)

UNDERAPPRECIATED?

Let me begin by saying, I have no right to complain; indeed, I am not complaining. It would never have occurred to me to argue (in public at least) that a particular paper of mine was under-cited, even worse ignored. But when the editor of this volume invited me to contribute, and shared with me his aims for the volume, I started to think, and from the thinking arose a few key issues whose consideration I thought might be of interest, even use, to others, especially younger scholars setting out on their careers. The lessons include: (1) Should you follow what science tells you is the interesting and worthwhile research question, and pursue that in glorious isolation, with no glance at the current fads and fashions of scholarship, or

(2) do you acknowledge, and give in to, the power of the Zeitgeist, understanding that timing is everything if your work is to have impact, and you are to have a career (and gain tenure)?

THE PAPER IN QUESTION

In 1987 I published a paper with the late Jos Jaspars entitled "Covariation and causal attribution: A logical model of the intuitive analysis of variance." It appeared in the *Journal of Personality and Social Psychology*, acknowledged as the leading outlet in our field, as indicated by its citation impact. I wrote the paper, as much as anything, as a posthumous tribute to my supervisor, who had died tragically young just a couple of years after I gained my doctorate. I knew he cared deeply about the "story" we had to tell, and he had had a major input to it, and a massive impact on me personally. He always believed, in a somewhat otherworldly way, that you should pursue questions of scientific merit, and try to come up with answers to satisfy your own intellectual curiosity, without worrying too much about anything else, least of all whether anyone would ever cite it.

The paper dealt with the rather arcane question of how lay perceivers combine different aspects of information in reaching a "causal attribution"—in short, how they decided to attribute a known effect to one or more possible causes. Indeed, when I look back at the issues now, I think "arcane" is a polite term. It all seems terribly dry and dull, and a long way from my current interests, which focus on real-world prejudice and intergroup conflict.

In a classic paper Harold Kelley (1967) had proposed that perceivers use three kinds of information, based on a lay version of J. S. Mill's "method of difference," to arrive at a causal conclusion: *consensus* (information about whether an effect was unique to one person or occurred in other people too), *consistency* (information about whether the effect occurred on only one occasion or had occurred on other occasions in the past), and *distinctiveness* (information about whether the effect was unique to one "entity" or occurred across other entities too). In Kelley's covariation model, an effect was attributable to a cause with which it covaried, a condition that was present when the effect was present, and absent when the effect was absent.

Leslie McArthur (now Zebrowitz) developed the elegant paradigm for testing this idea in 1972, and this became the standard for all subsequent studies on what came to be known as Kelley's "cube" model of attribution. This involved, simply, first presenting experimental subjects with an effect—for instance, "John laughed at the comedian." Then, in subsequent sentences, subjects received three pieces of information, each one designating a "high" or "low" level of consensus, consistency, and distinctiveness information. For example: "Almost everyone else laughed at the comedian" (high consensus); "John had not laughed at the comedian in the past" (low consistency); and "John did not laugh at any other comedian" (high distinctiveness). In McArthur's paradigm each of the three kinds of information could be "low" or "high," thus yielding a 2 (consensus: high vs. low) × 2 (consistency: high vs. low) × 2 (distinctiveness: high vs. low) analysis of variance (ANOVA) design, which resulted in eight different combinations or "patterns" of information. McArthur herself, and all subsequent authors, focused on the main effects in this ANOVA model, and for a long time researchers argued about which type of information had the greatest causal impact.

What was new about our model was that it was the first to emphasize that it was *patterns* of consensus, consistency, and distinctiveness that mattered, not main effects. We proposed that for each causal quandary (e.g., "Why did John laugh at the comedian"?) the lay perceiver could, and should, use all three pieces of information available and consider each potential single or multiple cause (e.g., was it something about the person? something about the situation? something about the person *and* situation? and so on). The subject's task was, in effect, we proposed, to test whether each potential single (or joint) cause was a necessary or sufficient "condition" for the occurrence of the effect. We demonstrated that for seven of the eight patterns our "logical model" highlighted what the perceiver (if logical and philosophically sophisticated) should identify as the cause, and moreover this model accounted well for the actual patterns of lay attribution.

WAS THE PAPER *UNDER*-CITED, AND IF SO WHY?

Logically, if I am to argue that our 1987 paper was *under*-cited, I should have some criterion in mind: How much should it have been cited? Before choosing to write about this paper I, of course, checked its citations. At the time of writing it had received 62 citations (according to Google Scholar). I emphasize, once again, that I don't really have much to complain about here; if all my papers were cited this often, I would probably be happy. Yet, by comparison, another paper I published in the same flagship journal, just two years earlier, had received 100 citations (Hewstone & Ward, 1985), despite it also dealing with attribution. Why?

I do still think the 1987 paper was elegant, a fact I attribute completely to the late, great Jos Jaspars, a brilliant thinker. Yet its timing was wrong, and the Zeitgeist had moved on. When I started out as a doctoral student at Oxford in 1978, working on attribution with Jaspars, a fellow member of the social group, Michael Argyle, told me in his inimitable style, "Ah! attribution . . . well, I've just come back from the USA, and learned that attribution theory is dead; wouldn't do that if I were you." And essentially he was right, in a way. As Jones (1985) pointed out, changing fashions in social psychology can be described as "bandwagons and sinking ships" (p. 54); the heyday of attribution theory was the late 1960s to the late 1970s, and I was arriving just a bit too late for the party. By failing, as a graduate student, to jump from sinking ship to bandwagon, I was, unwittingly, potentially passing up on any number of citations. It is instructive that the 1985 paper was on attribution theory and intergroup relations, the latter being a topic that was about to become a bandwagon.

I am also somewhat to blame myself, I suppose. Poor Jos was no longer around to develop the work and push the paper. But I chose to leave the topic of attribution patterns behind, preferring to extend the ideas of the second half of my thesis (where I linked attribution and intergroup relations) and devote almost all my research energies to the study of stereotyping, prejudice, and conflict. If I was not going to continue this line of work (and, of course, cite the paper), I could hardly complain if others failed to do so.

Finally, other models of causal attribution were published, some even more elegant than ours, and increasingly the area comprised just a few dedicated and uncompromising "attributionists," whose work seemed no longer to interest the majority of social psychologists. As my friend Wolfgang Stroebe once remarked to me, "You should title your next attribution paper 'Flogging a dead horse, or flogging a horse dead?'"

JE NE REGRETTE RIEN

In some confusion, having received Michael Argyle's devastating prognosis of my thesis topic, I went to see Jos Jaspars and asked him if he thought I should give up my current research questions and change to another area. I have never forgotten the calm, reasonable way he explained to me the importance of finding, and then trying to solve, interesting intellectual puzzles, and not worrying too much about popularity contests. But was he right?

Complex models of causal attribution turned out to be a wonderful topic to study as a graduate student; one could do lots of "neat" experiments, one could quite easily manipulate experimental variables of interest, and best of all, it taught me to think conceptually about quite complex issues. However, it also taught me to theorize, and not merely experiment, and this too was of enduring value in my career.

So the moral of my story is that "Timing is everything . . . at least in ensuring impact." I still like to think that the attribution paper brought things together in a way that was creative, but since the Zeitgeist in social psychology had moved on, its impact was necessarily limited. What, then, is the take-home point for others? Consider the advice of my two professors at Oxford. Was Jos Jaspars correct to urge me to follow the science, and my heart? Or was Michael Argyle right, judiciously advising me to think about the ebb and flow in the discipline, and the power of the Zeitgeist to dictate career decisions, indeed careers?

Thinking about this personal history, all these years later, I realize how fortunate I have been. It could have all gone terribly wrong. As it was, I did my spell as a player of what the author Hermann Hesse called "the glass-bead game." I devoted myself to the *vita contemplativa* and learned an enormous amount from that focus on the pure pursuit of intellectually challenging questions. But we now live in a world increasingly dominated by citation indices of "research impact" and the need to attract external research funding, which should have some benefit to wider society. It would be a brave adviser today who would tell his or her students that they could, or should, ignore the currents of research popularity. This also raises the question of when people should resist the tendency of social psychologists just to move on. Social psychology itself is full of illustrations of how slavish yielding to majority influence can be dysfunctional, and how minorities tend to trigger creative thinking. I have no special words of wisdom to offer here, but a cautious path would appear to be one that was not totally invested in an area that was deemed to be going out of fashion. Perhaps one should have one eye on scholarly pursuit, and the other eye on future employment (and therefore citation impact) as the one may come to a screeching halt—without the other.

REFERENCES

Hewstone, M., & Jaspars, J. (1987). Covariation and causal attribution: A logical model of the intuitive analysis of variance. *Journal of Personality and Social Psychology, 53*, 663–672.

Hewstone, M., & Ward, C. (1985). Ethnocentrism and causal attribution in Southeast Asia. *Journal of Personality and Social Psychology, 48*, 614–623.

Jones, E. E. (1985). Major developments in social psychology during the past four decades. In G. Lindzey & E. Aronson (Eds.), *Handbook of social psychology* (Vol. 1, pp. 47–108, 3rd ed.). New York: Random House.

Kelley, H. H. (1967). Attribution theory in social psychology. In D. Levine (Ed.), *Nebraska Symposium on Motivation* (Vol. 15, pp. 192–240). Lincoln: University of Nebraska Press.

McArthur, L. A. (1972). The how and what of why: Some determinants and consequences of causal attribution. *Journal of Personality and Social Psychology, 22*, 171–193.

REX A. WRIGHT, University of Alabama at Birmingham

Motivational When Motivational Wasn't Cool

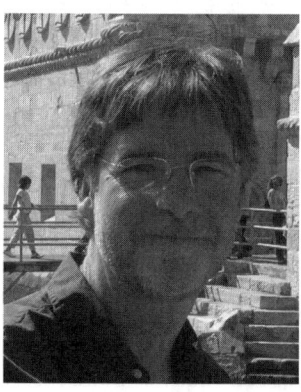

Jack Brehm was invited to contribute to this volume, but died before he got the chance. Thus, I am writing in his stead. Jack's career was dedicated to understanding social motivational processes. He persisted in pursuing motivational themes even when his pursuits conflicted with (e.g., cognitive) trends in social psychology and the field of psychology as a whole. He also persisted when his efforts yielded modest payoff in terms of academic currencies such as publications and grants. Any social psychologist worth his or her professional salt is aware of Jack's profound contributions in the areas of cognitive dissonance and psychological reactance. However, many are unaware that these are only two of four "grand ideas" with which Jack was associated. One additional grand idea was his theory of motivational intensity (Brehm & Self, 1989); the other was its sister theory of emotional intensity (Brehm, 1999). Although these last ideas are less well known than the earlier ones, it is arguable that they constitute Jack's most brilliant contributions to psychological science. Consequently, I will discuss them briefly here.

In discussing Jack's motivation intensity theory, I will focus on the theory's subjective implications because they have been especially subject to neglect. Jack began developing this theory toward the end of his time at Duke University. He refined and ultimately moved beyond it once he moved to the University of Kansas. The first written sketch is seen in an early (and unfunded) grant proposal that outlined what Jack then identified as his theory of motivational suppression (Brehm, 1975). The suppression analysis concerned motivational arousal, construed broadly ("energization"), and posited a mechanism that allows such arousal to occur only to the degree that it is needed. Two key propositions were that energy is in fact needed (1) only when a potential outcome (incentive) is possible to obtain and worth obtaining, and (2) only to the extent that imminent or ongoing instrumental (required) behavior is difficult to execute. Together, these propositions implied that motivational arousal should vary non-monotonically with the difficulty of imminent or ongoing behavior, first rising and then falling, with the fall occurring where success calls for more than people can or will do. A third proposition was that feelings of need and desire to satisfy the motive driving behavior (e.g., the motive to obtain food) track motivational arousal levels. This suggested that just as motivational arousal should first rise and then fall with difficulty, so should felt need and desire.

To illustrate the effects described above, consider two "tweens" provided the chance to earn album downloads for their iPhones by playing peacefully for a full day. Peaceful play = one download apiece; even one fight = no downloads. In theory, experienced energy as well as felt need and desire for the album downloads should vary depending on the difficulty of the play challenge. If the tweens are highly compatible, in terms of personality, the challenge should be relatively easy and the tweens should experience little energy, need, and desire. If the tweens are not so compatible, the challenge should be more difficult and the tweens should experience increased energy, need, and desire so long as they view success as possible and worthwhile. If the tweens are incompatible to the point that they view success as excessively difficult—given the contingent benefit (i.e., the album downloads)—or impossible, energy, need, and desire should be low.

An interesting feature of the early suppression version of the motivation intensity theory is that it made no mention of effort. This is interesting because, insofar as the intensity theory has had an impact within the scientific community, it has had one chiefly serving as a model of effort, applied most often to predict physiological outcomes. People familiar with the theory frequently are surprised to learn that effort was incorporated into Jack's thinking somewhat after the fact, largely as the result of discussions with graduate students.

Later versions of the intensity theory that Jack developed assumed explicitly that people apply themselves more and less intensively to behavioral challenges and that motivational arousal corresponds to their degree of application. They also de-emphasized the hypothesized suppression mechanism and emphasized an important distinction between "cool" cognitive incentive appraisals and "warm" affective incentive appraisals. Regarding the distinction, later versions posited that people can maintain stable understandings of how much (resource investment) potential positive and negative outcomes are worth while simultaneously experiencing variations in felt need or desire to attain and avoid those outcomes, respectively. Thus, for example, a woman might maintain a consistent intellectual assessment of how much a car is worth across a week of purchase deliberation, but—during that period—vary in how much she *wants* the car. In theory, the woman's intellectual assessment should determine how much need and desire she could experience, whereas difficulty factors should determine the need and desire that she actually experiences. Jack's distinction between cognition and affect in motivational contexts was especially insightful and addressed the difficult question of how incentive appraisals can vary with effort and motivational arousal as well as determine the upper limit of these outcomes.

Data relevant to the subjective implications of the intensity theory were collected for more than a decade. Early student collaborators were Tom Pyszczynski, Linda Silka, Sheldon Solomon, and Challenger Vought. Later collaborators included Paul Biner, Luis Esqueda, Carol Ford, Jeff Greenberg, Tom Hill, Bruce Roberson, Elizabeth Self, Miho Toi, and me. As motivation intensity theory evolved, it moved from being discussed as Jack's theory of motivational suppression to being discussed as his energization theory of motivation to eventually being discussed in motivation intensity terms. Naturally, studies did not always work. However, as a group, they generated a remarkable degree of support.

To illustrate, studies of felt need and desire documented repeatedly the implication that people should find positive outcomes especially attractive (i.e., desirable) when the outcomes are moderately difficult to secure. They also documented the mirror implication that people should find negative outcomes especially aversive (undesirable) when the outcomes are moderately difficult to avoid. As expected, difficulty effects on incentive appraisals were found to be moderated by factors that should determine cool cognitive incentive appraisals (e.g., the objective value of the incentive) and to be present when action was imminent, but not when it was completed or to occur at a distant point in the future. Also as expected, the difficulty effects were found to be associated with corresponding effects on physiological indices of energization, such as changes in blood pressure. Notably, the need and desire studies employed an array of incentives and tasks, confirming that findings were not limited to particular procedures. They also ruled out alternative processes such as reactance, cognitive dissonance, and expectancy of success by controlling factors that would allow those processes to operate.

Despite the richness of its reasoning and the strong picture conveyed by the body of relevant evidence, the motivation intensity theory drew little attention at the time and has drawn only modest attention to this day. As noted previously, to the degree the theory has been recognized, it has been so as a model of effort, which is well removed from the theory's first purpose. Jack was puzzled by the muted response, but in his signature low-key fashion, not greatly bothered by it. He did science not to attract attention, but rather to acquire an improved understanding of phenomena that interested him. Driven by this latter purpose, Jack pressed ahead.

EMOTION INTENSITY

Somewhere in the early 1990s, Jack had what he might have described as an epiphany. His new idea rested on a common assumption: that affective components of motivation (i.e., feelings of need and desire) function to facilitate, or urge, appropriate action. Jack reasoned that if this is true, need and desire might vary not with instrumental task difficulty alone, but rather with *any* factor that opposes them or the action that they are urging. So long as a motive is possible to satisfy and worth satisfying, felt need and desire can function effectively only if they are great enough to overcome (1) any (mental or physical) difficulty that might be involved, and (2) any other opposing force, or deterrent, that exists. An example of a deterrent other than difficulty would be the price of an item available for sale. Although a progressively higher price would not call for progressively higher effort, it would increasingly oppose the action being urged (i.e., purchase) and could be argued to oppose feelings of need and desire themselves. As a result, the progressively higher price should lead to increased feelings of need and desire to a point and then cause the feelings to drop to a chronically low level. This insight led Jack to wonder whether he and his students might have been too narrow in focusing on difficulty over the years. It also led him to wonder whether a broader statement might be made about affective system function.

Once Jack had his deterrence insight, it took him little time to develop his final theory, that of emotional intensity. The theory assumed that emotions are motivational states insofar as they urge action (e.g., flight). It also involved the construct of emotional deterrence, defining an emotional deterrent as any factor that opposes either an emotion or the action urged by it. One example of an emotional deterrent would be a joyful event occurring to someone who has been prompted by a loss to experience sadness. The joyful event would be contrary to (i.e., oppose) the sad feeling. Additional examples would be strength in an opponent against whom one is urged by anger to aggress and reticence in a partner with whom one is urged by lust to have sex. Strength would oppose attack and reticence would oppose physical intimacy. The theory's core proposition was that emotional intensity varies directly not with the magnitude of an emotional stimulus, as most people would assume, but rather with the magnitude of emotion deterrence. Further, the relation between emotion intensity and deterrence should be non-monotonic, with intensity rising with deterrence so long as the motive relevant to the emotion is stronger than the deterrent and then showing a sharp drop. Thus, for example, reticence in a potential sex partner should intensify ardor up to the point that its strength exceeds the strength of the motive to have sex and then cause ardor to drop.

Jack spent his last years investigating this analysis. Student collaborators of special note were Beverly Brummett, Kathleen Fuegen, Anca Miron, and Paul Silvia. Like studies conducted to test the implications of Jack's motivation intensity analysis, studies conducted to test the implications of his emotion intensity analysis did not always work. However, many did, and collectively the studies produced a compelling body of support. For example, the studies documented repeatedly the implication that a positive emotion (e.g., happiness) could be increased and then decreased by the presentation of increasingly powerful unpleasant (e.g., graduation requirement) information. They also documented the implication that a negative emotion could be altered via the presentation of increasingly powerful pleasant information and confirmed the theory's predictive utility in special social circumstances, such as ones involving love. Nonetheless, the theory attracted limited notice for the better part of this period, and Jack died uncertain whether more than a handful of colleagues and students would ever "get it."

DISCOVERY AND A LESSON

To end favorably, there is reason to believe that investigators might be discovering Jack's emotion theory. Citations of relevant articles are up and the informal "buzz" in private discussions appears to be increasing. Jack would have been pleased, but more for the scientific community than for himself. Jack understood that first-tier ideas do not necessarily "rise to the top." With this in mind, he focused on the process—the scientific ride. In doing so, he allowed himself to enjoy his progress and remain encouraged even when others did not see what he saw. There was marvelous wisdom in Jack's focus, and that wisdom might be the best lesson to be taken from this tale.

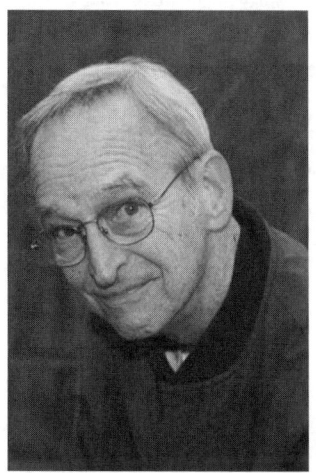

Jack Brehm, 1928–2009

AUTHOR NOTE

I am grateful to Sharon Brehm and Anca Miron for reviewing early drafts of this piece.

REFERENCES

Brehm, J. W. (1975). *A theory of motivational suppression.* Unpublished grant proposal, University of Kansas.

Brehm, J. W. (1999). The intensity of emotion. *Personality and Social Psychology Review, 3,* 2–22.

Brehm, J. W., & Self, E. (1989). The intensity of motivation. In M. R. Rozenweig & L. W. Porter (Eds.), *Annual Review of Psychology* (pp. 109–131). Palo Alto: Annual Reviews, Inc.

MARK R. LEARY, Duke University

Does Impression Management Have an Image Problem?

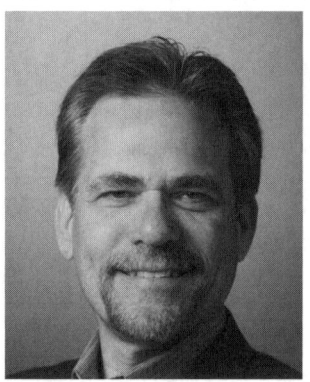

A few years ago, while sorting through a box of personal memorabilia, I stumbled upon the personal statement that I had written for my application to graduate school. Reading what I had written about myself and my professional goals evoked a bit of a shock. Not only did I realize that my research over the past 30 years had borne almost no connection to the claims I had made about my intellectual interests at the time that I applied to graduate school, but I also fully appreciated for the first time how fortunate I was that several programs had decided to accept me in spite of the overblown verbiage in my rather clueless personal statement. Had I been making the decision, I'm not sure that I would have accepted me on the basis of what I had written.

After weighing my options, I had decided to attend the University of Florida to work with Barry Schlenker because he was one of only three social psychologists, along with E. E. "Ned" Jones and James Tedeschi, who had an ongoing program of research on self-presentation. I could not have known it when I started graduate school, but my work with Barry defined my career and paved the way for my own research and writing on the ways in which people's behavior is influenced by their concerns with how they are perceived, evaluated, and accepted by others.

Although the rambling statement on my application contained no mention of either social interactions or self-presentation, I decided that I was interested primarily in how people relate to each other in face-to-face interactions and specifically in how their desires that others view them in particular ways—and not view them in other ways—influence their behavior and emotions. Barry did not think that self-presentation was at the root of every interpersonal behavior, but given that people can rarely afford to disregard what others think of them, he insisted that the possibility of self-presentational influences always be considered. However, I soon began to detect that much of the field did not share his conviction that self-presentational influences were nearly always operating, and in fact, many social psychologists held an entrenched bias against self-presentational explanations of behavior. Impression management seemed to have an image problem.

A few years before I started graduate school, Tedeschi, Schlenker, and Bonoma (1971) had suggested in a controversial article that many phenomena that had been explained in terms of cognitive dissonance were due more to people's concerns with appearing inconsistent to other people than with intrapsychic pressures arising from cognitive inconsistency per se, a claim that had been supported by a number of experiments. In fact, the first study of self-presentation in which I became involved as a graduate student was one such study (Schlenker, Forsyth, Leary, & Miller, 1980; Study 3). The results of this research showed that people who had performed a behavior contrary to their attitudes showed dissonance-like effects primarily when they had reason to think that others would perceive them as inconsistent or immoral for acting in a counter-attitudinal fashion. Pure cognitive inconsistency did not produce the effects, as dissonance theory would predict.

As a graduate student, I had naïvely expected this line of work to offer a dramatic challenge to dissonance theory, but in general, self-presentational reinterpretations of dissonance effects were met with resounding silence. Indeed, only 10 publications ever cited the Schlenker et al. (1980) article (which was published in the *Journal of Personality and Social Psychology*), and only two of the citing articles involved a peer-reviewed article published in English by someone who was not a co-author of the original paper. Furthermore, with two exceptions, both of them also involving co-authors of the article, I have not seen the self-presentational interpretation of dissonance effects even mentioned in any social psychology textbook. Perhaps the reaction was predictable: Many researchers in the 1960s and 1970s had devoted a great deal of effort to the study of dissonance-based phenomena, and they were understandably not enthused to be told that the picture was more complicated than they had thought or, worse, that they were possibly wrong.

Yet, the issue appears to run deeper than resistance to a perspective that conflicted with a particular revered theory. With each article, chapter, and book that I've published on the topic of self-presentation, I've sensed that the self-presentational perspective is not as appreciated by social psychologists as one would expect given the pervasiveness and strength of the processes involved and the variety of research findings that support it. Social psychologists no longer seem antagonistic to self-presentation—merely uninterested, rarely considering self-presentational explanations except perhaps as a last resort when some other theory cannot explain their pattern of results.

At one point, I thought that I might be able to promote interest in impression management with a comprehensive literature review that was framed within a conceptual framework that distinguished between factors that influence the degree to which people are motivated to impression-manage and factors that determine the content of the impressions that they try to make (Leary & Kowalski, 1990). This article has been reasonably well cited overall—but not in mainline social psychology journals. In nearly 20 years, it was cited only ten times in the *Journal of Personality and Social Psychology* and six times in *Personality and Social Psychology Bulletin,* and about half of those citations were by another researcher who has had a longstanding interest in self-presentation. As another indication of the field's lack of enthusiasm for self-presentation, of more than 500 symposia that have been scheduled at the annual meetings of the Society for Personality and Social Psychology during the past 10 years, only one has focused specifically on self-presentation.

In contrast, fields other than social psychology seem to appreciate the self-presentational perspective more than social psychologists do. In particular, work in management and organizational behavior has drawn heavily on self-presentational concepts, as has research in sport and exercise psychology. In addition, a later article that examined self-presentational aspects of health risk behavior (Leary, Tchividjian, & Kraxberger, 1994) garnered a good deal of attention among health psychologists in how people's concerns with their social image can lead them to engage in unhealthy behaviors.

Social psychologists' general lack of interest in self-presentation puzzles me. Not only are most people pervasively concerned with what other people think of them, but they do many things to make desired impressions on other people. How people fare in life depends, in part, on being perceived in certain ways and in avoiding making undesired impressions, so it is not surprising that self-presentational influences pervade human life. Even when their primary goal in a social encounter is not to make an impression, people usually pursue their focal goals in ways that do not taint their images in other people's eyes. So, why aren't social psychologists more amenable to self-presentational explanations of human behavior and devoting more time and effort to studying the complexities of impression management?

One reason might be that the general notion that people are broadly concerned with what other people think of them and sometimes try to convey particular impressions of themselves to others is not a particularly profound insight. Everyone knows it to be true, even if many of us decry the emphasis that some people place on their public images. As a result, at the most basic level, there's no "gee-whiz" factor in self-presentational theory or research that makes people sit up and take notice. Of course, plenty of mundane, commonsensical phenomena have been widely studied by social psychologists, so topics do not need a high gee-whiz factor to garner attention. For example, I doubt that anyone was surprised to learn that people aggress more when they are frustrated or regard members of their own groups more favorably than members of outgroups, yet those effects have been widely studied and discussed. Furthermore, the fact that a phenomenon is not surprising or counterintuitive does not mean that it is not important or doesn't help to explain a great deal of variability in thought, emotion, and behavior. In fact, the opposite may be true: The most powerful influences on human behavior may be the least surprising because their power is obvious to everyone.

Perhaps part of the problem is that most experimental studies (including many of mine) have not captured the complexity of people's self-presentations in everyday life, so neither the designs nor the findings are very snazzy or memorable. The antecedent variables that have been studied—such as other people's values, social pressures, or one's own self-concept—are relatively straightforward, as are the dependent variables, which mostly involve self-ratings on questionnaires that participants believe will be seen by other people. In everyday self-presentation, people exclude information from their self-presentations that would under-mine their image, but participants in research are more or less forced to describe themselves on particular attributes. Furthermore, a great deal of real-life self-presentation involves shadings and nuances that are difficult to capture in experimental settings. On top of that, in their daily lives, people often must juggle many images and many audiences simultaneously, whereas most studies involve only one or two images and a single target. Put simply, laboratory studies of self-presentation often reflect only a pale and impoverished version of the complex, dynamic process that occurs in people's everyday lives. Perhaps it is notewor-thy that studies that examine the effects of self-presentational processes on other phenomena—such as risk-taking, unflattering self-presentations, or moral behavior—typically use more interesting paradigms, and these studies tend to attract more attention.

Another possible reason that self-presentational explanations are invoked so rarely is that, despite the fact that social psychology ostensibly focuses on the effects of other people and social contexts on behavior, the field relies heavily on intrapsychic explanations. As noted earlier, people's efforts to deal with behavioral inconsistency have been attributed to an intrapsychic motive to avoid cognitive dissonance rather than to their desire to be viewed as consistent to other people because being perceived as inconsistent engenders negative evaluations and inter-personal problems. Similarly, many self-enhancement effects that have been attrib-uted to an internal need for self-esteem can be explained in terms of people's efforts to be evaluated positively by other people; in general, people appear to be more concerned with what other people think of them than with what they think of themselves. I am not suggesting that people are not sometimes motivated to main-tain certain cognitive or emotional states, but rather that social psychologists often invoke intrapsychic explanations for behavior even when interpersonal explanations, including self-presentation, may be more plausible.

Finally, acknowledging the pervasive impact of self-presentation opens a very large can of worms for scientists who study social behavior. Once one admits that people are rarely unconcerned with others' judgments of them, one must acknowledge that many research findings might reflect people's efforts to be seen in particular ways rather than whatever process one is purportedly investigating. The intrusion of self-presentational concerns into research settings is typically regarded as a methodological problem, which it often is, yet the fact that researchers are so concerned that participants in their studies might be impression-managing suggests that the social psychological phenomenon under investigation might have a strong self-presentational component in everyday life. One researcher's confound is another's primary interest.

People's behavior is influenced by countless factors, of which their desire to be perceived in particular ways by other people is only one. No one has seriously suggested that all human behavior is self-presentational, although some critics have leveled that charge. But given that self-presentational concerns arguably rank among the most potent interpersonal influences on social behavior, one might expect social psychology to be far more deeply involved in studying these processes than it is. Despite the efforts of a small number of researchers, including myself, the topic of impression management remains underappreciated by many social psychologists.

REFERENCES

Leary, M. R., & Kowalski, R. M. (1990). Impression management: A literature review and two-component model. *Psychological Bulletin, 107,* 34–47.

Leary, M. R., Tchividjian, L. R., & Kraxberger, B. E. (1994). Self-presentation can be hazardous to your health: Impression management and health risk. *Health Psychology, 13,* 461–470.

Schlenker, B. R., Forsyth, D. R., Leary, M. R., & Miller, R. S. (1980). A self-presentational analysis of the effects of incentives on attitude change following counterattitudinal behavior. *Journal of Personality and Social Psychology, 39,* 553–577.

Tedeschi, J. T., Schlenker, B. R., & Bonoma, T. V. (1971). Cognitive dissonance: Private ratiocination or public spectacle? *American Psychologist, 26,* 685–695.

DELROY L. PAULHUS, University of British Columbia

Dynamic Complexity Theory: Eclipsed by a Revolution

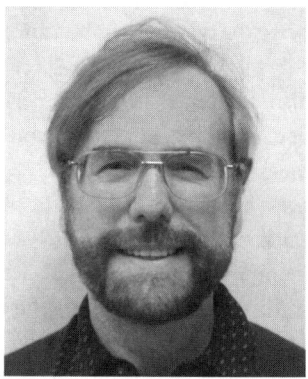

Timing is of the essence. Sure, an argument can be made for insight and creativity in science. But devoting one's efforts to a program of research that arrives D.O.A. is best avoided. The example I can offer from my career is the three-year swatch of time I spent developing dynamic complexity theory (Paulhus, 1987).

COGNITIVE COMPLEXITY

At the time, the historical trajectory seemed to be ripe for a process model of complexity. The evolution of work on cognitive complexity began with George Kelly and was elaborated via contributions from such names as Harvey, Hunt, Shroeder, Streufert, and Driver. In the 1970s, this line of thought culminated in integrative complexity theory as articulated by Peter Suedfeld and Phil Tetlock. Those researchers did address certain forms of fluctuations in complexity, but I felt that the dynamics had not been fully explored. I was also optimistic that these ideas had the potential for elaboration into a broader theory of personality.

The most direct inspiration for my dynamic perspective was a paper by Michael Driver (1962). Although published only as a technical report, and relatively unheralded as a consequence, Driver's paper demonstrated a fascinating link between stress and social perception. In a rich simulation of international warfare, participants played the role of world leaders. At several points of the simulation, participants were asked to rate their perceptions of the countries represented by the other "leaders." In early ratings, participants exhibited relatively complex perceptions. At a key point, however, participants were subjected to a stress manipulation in the form of an imminent war. As stress increased, participants tended to reduce their perceptual space to two dimensions: evaluation and potency. Driver concluded that world leaders threatened with war are likely to simplify their world view. Under such conditions, it is essential to focus on two characteristics of other countries: Are they friendly (*evaluation*) and are they are powerful (*potency*)? Less-important perceptual dimensions will drop out, thereby magnifying the perceived importance of the two critical decision dimensions.

To me, those results hinted at an optimal mechanism for linking person perception to decision behavior. The notion was reminiscent of *graceful degradation,* a concept borrowed from computer systems jargon: The shutdown sequence in an optimal computer system is designed to ensure that essential processes shut down last. I suspected that reductions in cognitive complexity under stress also followed a systematic order: The last dimensions to degrade should be those that (a) are most elementary and (b) can protect the integrity of the system as a whole. When I applied graceful degradation to human decision-making, a broader psychological theory fell into place.

DYNAMIC COMPLEXITY THEORY

The theory comprised five propositions. First, emotional stressors tend to reduce the cognitive complexity of interpersonal perceptions. Second, the ordering of these reductions is such that evaluation and potency become more salient. Third, the effects of stress are mediated by arousal that precedes the processing of other information. Fourth, the enhanced role of evaluation and potency act to protect the individual from the threat. Fifth, individual differences in trait complexity moderate the changes in complexity, and therefore the effectiveness of the threat. My review paper (Paulhus, 1987) offered a wealth of supportive data, but only one journal article ensued (Paulhus & Lim, 1991).

In one study, participants were asked to rate the similarities of a subset of their acquaintances. Soft versus loud white noise was used to manipulate arousal during the rating task. Under loud white noise, participants showed a reduction in the complexity of the similarity space. Moreover, the evaluation dimension (which was evident in the perceptual space of all participants) was even more predominant in the social perceptions of those participants subjected to loud noise. The potency dimension also remained evident under such stressful conditions. A total of 10 studies replicated and extended this result to support all five propositions.

Automatic vs. Controlled Processing

During the same era, a distinction between automatic and controlled processing (ACP) entered mainstream social psychology with a review chapter by John Bargh. Most of the reviewed research came directly from the field of cognitive psychology: Only a handful of the empirical studies to that date were social psychological in content. To simplify the distinction, controlled processes are effortful, whereas automatic processes can operate with minimal cognitive resources.

The ACP distinction provided a powerful notion with wide heuristic applications. As pointed out by colleagues and reviewers alike, the propositions of dynamic complexity theory could also be handled by the ACP theory. For example, emotional stress undermines controlled processing, thereby forcing (simpler) automatic processes to control cognition as well as behavior.

Needless to say, the impact of ACP has been deep and broad. Moreover, a spate of other two-factor theories ensued. All of them addressed what appears to be a qualitative shift in the nature of cognitive processing under stress. *Sic transit gloria*: No longer could I argue for any special contribution from dynamic complexity theory.

LESSONS

Looking back, I still believe that dynamic complexity theory is among my most creative and defensible efforts. Nonetheless, the ideas were eclipsed by a revolutionary and more powerful framework. Not all was lost: The intangible benefits of theory-building carried over to my subsequent (and more recognized) work on apparently distant topics such as self-presentation. For example, my latest arguments regarding the diversity of self-presentation variables recommend a narrowed focus on two primary themes: communion and agency (Paulhus & Trapnell, 2008). These two themes bear an uncanny resemblance to evaluation and potency, respectively.

Based on other essays in this book, my experience is not unique. With well-deserved humility, I offer two lessons to more junior researchers. The first is to anticipate scientific revolutions, and in so doing, avoid having one's hard-wrought ideas eclipsed. There is little point to persevering on work relegated to the shadows. A second (and less insipid) lesson is that the same data can often be couched within more than one conceptual framework. Often the differences may appear to be merely semantic—that is, old wine in new bottles. But one's choice of framework has pivotal consequences for the subsequent impact of one's research.

REFERENCES

Driver, M. J. (1962). *Conceptual structure and group processes in an inter-nation simulation. Part one: the perception of simulated nations* (Report 1962-15). Princeton, NJ: Educational Testing Service.

Paulhus, D. L. (1987). A dynamic complexity theory of personality processes. *Manuscript rejected by Psychological Review*.

Paulhus, D. L., & Lim, D. T. K. (1994). Arousal and evaluative extremity in social judgments: A dynamic complexity model. *European Journal of Social Psychology, 24*, 89–99.

Paulhus, D. L., & Trapnell, P. D. (2008). Self-presentation: An agency-communion framework. In O. P. John, R. W. Robins, & L. A. Pervin (Eds.), *Handbook of personality psychology* (pp. 492–517). New York: Guilford.

PART III

Methods and Innovations

ROBERT B. CIALDINI, Arizona State University

Littering as an Unobtrusive Measure of Political Attitudes: Messy but Clean

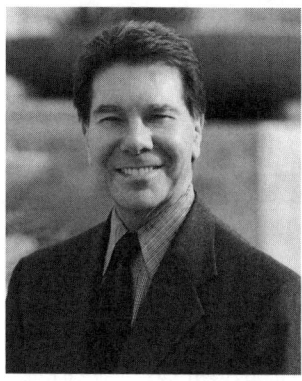

The great German physicist Werner Heisenberg won a Nobel Prize for his role in developing the modern science of quantum mechanics, from which came the famous Heisenberg Principle. According to this principle, which is said to govern all of science, the act of measuring something alters that thing at least slightly. For instance, we've all no doubt recognized that our responses change when someone is seen to be observing and recording them. Of course, scientists studying others' attitudes want to record them in their truest, least altered form. Consequently, they frequently rely on certain proven methods for reducing the impact of the act of measurement on their data.

One such method is to gauge an attitude by using unobtrusive (covert) means to measure it. Rather than asking for a self-report of the attitude at issue, a researcher employing an unobtrusive assessment may record an attitude-relevant behavior that experimental participants don't know is being recorded and then infer the participants' attitude from it. In this way, many of the potential measurement distortions associated with self-reports (e.g., demand characteristics, self-presentational pressures) can be reduced. For instance, if researchers want to know the attitude in a certain neighborhood toward racial integration, they might record the percentage of people there who will mail a "lost" letter secretly placed on the street and addressed to the Council For Racial Integration. The more letters that are mailed, the more favorable is the presumed attitude. Scientists using this *lost letter technique* (Milgram, Mann, & Harter, 1965) have been able to gauge public attitudes toward a variety of sensitive topics such as abortion, communism, and homosexuality.

In general, researchers have found that these covert techniques are more accurate than self-report measures only when people have a good reason to be less than honest about their true feelings—for example, when they want to appear more fairminded or unprejudiced than they actually are. Under these circumstances, covert techniques are preferred because they are more non-reactive than self-reports; that is, using them to record a response is less likely to distort the response. When there is no good reason for people to hide their feelings, however, self-reports are usually preferred because they inquire about attitudes more directly.

LITTERING AS AN UNOBTRUSIVE MEASURE OF ATTITUDE

Some years ago, my graduate student at the time, Don Baumann, and I accidentally hit upon an unobtrusive measure that had not been documented before (Cialdini & Baumann, 1981). The measure came to our attention while we were conducting a study of the conditions affecting the decision to litter in a public place. Participants leaving a convenience store were handed a flier advocating driver safety. We noticed that any littering of the flier occurred away from the view of the person who was dispensing the fliers but not necessarily away from the view of other persons in the area. When questioned regarding this tendency, participants indicated that they had not wished to discard the handbill—and to appear to disagree with its message—in front of someone who was obviously committed to that message. Within such an explanation, we realized, was the suggestion that littering could be seen as a measure of attitude.

That is, because of a desire to disassociate oneself from disliked materials, the act of retaining or discarding a printed message might reflect affective positivity or negativity toward that message. In order to test the possibility, we performed an initial experiment to determine whether littering had merit as a valid measure of attitude. Our prediction was that retention of a printed message would indicate a favorable opinion of the message content, whereas littering of the message would indicate an unfavorable opinion. We tested the prediction in the context of the 1976 Jimmy Carter–Gerald Ford presidential election. Our research assistants placed fliers advocating the candidacy of either Carter or Ford on the car windshields of voters who had parked at one of nine voting locations and then proceeded into the location to cast a vote. Our expectation was that, upon returning to their cars and encountering one or another of the fliers, Carter voters would more frequently retain Carter fliers and litter Ford fliers than would Ford voters. We also conducted an exit poll of the drivers—which later vote counts proved to be highly accurate—that allowed us to identify which voters preferred Carter or Ford.

The results supported our prediction in that, among those who littered, 63% had received a flier advocating their nonfavored candidate and 37% had received a flier advocating their favored candidate. Among those who retained the flier, the pattern was reversed: 67% had received a flier advocating their favored candidate and 33% their nonfavored candidate. Moreover, via our littering measure, we were able to predict the winner at each of the nine voting stations that we employed in our study well before the election results were announced.

WHEN IS LITTERING LIKELY TO BE A USEFUL MEASURE OF ATTITUDE?

Although we were pleased with the outcome, another aspect of our results informed us that there was no reason for attitude researchers to adopt our littering measure wholesale: Not only had littering patterns predicted the victor at all nine voting stations, so had our simple exit poll that asked participants to self-report which candidate had gotten their vote. We weren't surprised that a traditional, self-report survey would do as well as our littering measure in the election context we examined. Because the primary benefit of the littering index over more traditional measures of attitude lies in its unobtrusive and, therefore, nonreactive character, one should expect it to provide a more accurate assessment principally on controversial or sensitive topics. It is with such topics that direct survey and self-report procedures may be susceptible to the range of self-presentational pressures that lead to measurement distortions; see Greenwald, Poehlman, Uhlmann, and Banaji (2009) for recent verification of this contention. An unobtrusive measure like littering should minimize these pressures and, therefore, should only allow for a more representative estimate of attitude toward issues with large social desirability components (e.g., ethical, racial, sexual, or charitable issues).

To test these predictions, we conducted an experiment at Arizona State University in which participants' attitudes toward one of two issues were measured either by the littering procedure or by a direct survey question. The attitude issues concerned either support for the Equal Rights Amendment for women (large social desirability component) or support for the reinstatement of the recently discharged football coach (small social desirability component). Although both topics concerned issues of some currency on campus at the time of the experiment, only the ERA question could be construed as having a socially approved side within the university community. Favorability toward the ERA was the socially desirable response. Even though it seemed evident to us that the ERA issue was the more social desirability-laden of the two topics, we did not have empirical confirmation of that assumption. Therefore, we sought to separate the two topics more surely along the social desirability dimension by employing female experimenters, who were instructed to dress as a feminist might.[1] Thus, a female interviewer inquiring about the ERA could be seen to have a clear preference on the issue (in direction of favorability) but no such preference would be implied in the instance of the coach reinstatement. Our specific hypotheses, then, were that the littering and interview techniques would produce similar attitude patterns for the coach reinstatement topic but different patterns for the ERA topic, with the interview method generating more favorable responses for the ERA.

Participants were solitary males returning to one of three student parking lots in which all cars had previously received one of four windshield fliers. Two of the fliers concerned the ERA ("Support the Equal Rights Amendment" or "Oppose the Equal Rights Amendment"); the other two concerned the football coach's reinstatement ("Support the Reinstatement of Frank Kush" or "Oppose the Reinstatement of Frank Kush"). In the interview condition, as a participant entered the lot, he was approached by an experimenter carrying a clipboard. She inquired into the subject's opinion on one of the topics as follows:

> "Hello, I'm conducting a survey concerning the (Equal Rights Amendment/reinstatement of coach Frank Kush) issue. Could you tell me if you support or oppose the (Equal Rights Amendment/reinstatement of Frank Kush)?"

In the littering technique condition, an individual meeting the conditions defining a participant passed the experimenter but was not approached by her. The type of flier on his car and whether the subject littered or retained the flier were recorded from a distance.

Our predictions were confirmed. For the social desirability-laden ERA issue, 75% of the subjects responded favorably when measured by the interview procedure, while only 46% did so when measured by the littering technique. However, for the issue lacking in a large social desirability component (i.e., the football coach's reinstatement), the two measurement techniques produced nearly identical response distributions (58% versus 56%, respectively).

SUMMARY AND CONCLUSIONS

An initial study found that after voting in a presidential election, people were less likely to litter a handbill they found on the windshield of their cars if the handbill's message supported their favored candidate. In fact, before the official voting totals were announced, this measure correctly predicted the winning candidate at all nine of the voting locations where it was used—but so did a simple exit poll that asked people how they voted. Thus, when there was little reason for individuals to conceal their actual attitudes, this self-report measure was just as accurate as the covert one. However, in a follow-up study using the politically sensitive topic of increased women's rights, the pattern was quite different. When asked by a college-age female survey taker whether they supported or opposed the ERA, the great majority (75%) of male undergraduates voiced their support. But when attitude was measured covertly, by how likely male undergraduates were to litter a handbill that either supported or opposed this amendment, less than half (46%) appeared supportive.

The littering measure has a number of properties to recommend it for use in a variety of research contexts. First, the attitudes of preselected subjects may be assessed by providing specific individuals with a flier or handbill. Second, no complicated apparatus is required; therefore, the technique is both mobile and inexpensive. Third, the message format allows for more detailed and calibrated attitude statements than simple pro and con communications; that is, the handbill medium permits the presentation of a large range of subtly shaded positions. Finally, the technique may be used away from the laboratory or campus, thereby reducing demand artifacts.

A GENERAL QUALIFICATION

Despite the advantages of the littering technique, there is an important caveat to be recognized. The technique is unlikely to provide an accurate measure of the population distributions of pro versus anti attitudes on some topic when those individuals holding pro attitudes have a different base-rate tendency to litter than those holding anti attitudes. For example, if there were a good reason to believe that individuals favoring the legalization of gambling littered more, generally, that those opposing the legalization of gambling, the littering technique would be inadvisable as a means for assessing population attitudes on that issue. However, the necessary assumption of comparable base-rate response tendencies within the measured groups is hardly unique to the littering procedure, nor even to unobtrusive techniques. For instance, if one wished to measure accurately the attitude toward legalized gambling in a given population via the lost letter technique, one would need to assume that pro-gambling individuals have a disposition to help (by mailing a lost letter) comparable to that of anti-gambling individuals. Similarly, if the measurement device were a self-report or direct interview, it would be necessary to assume that pro- and anti-gambling advocates respond to surveys with equivalent degrees of honesty and accuracy.

In all, then, it appears that the littering technique offers a relatively convenient, inexpensive, valid, and nonreactive measure of attitude. Yet, it (along with the article that described it to the scientific community) has gone unnoticed and unused and, accordingly, has become a fitting candidate for this book. It's possible to speculate on why this might be the case. Of course, in the realm of speculation, causality is always uncertain. Still, I have a favored explanation: The timing was wrong. Our article and technique appeared in the lull of interest in non-reactive measures between their heyday in the 1960s, which featured the work of such luminaries as Milgram, Campbell, and McClelland, and the resurgence of that interest in modern examinations of implicit attitudes. If I am right, perhaps the timely exposure provided by this publication will change an appreciation gap into a mere appreciation lag. That would be great, as no investigator wants to see a favored finding—much like a favored attitude—tossed to the side of the road.

NOTE

1. No specific instructions were provided in this regard; rather, the experimenters were allowed to dress in ways defined by their own stereotypes and wardrobe closets. The result was a predominance of Levis, cotton, and khaki and an absence of skirts, dresses, and polyester.

REFERENCES

Cialdini, R. B., Baumann, D. J. (1981). Littering: A new unobtrusive measure of attitude. *Social Psychology Quarterly, 44*, 254–259.

Greenwald, A. G., Poehlman, T. A., Uhlman, E. L., & Banaji, M. B. (2009). Understanding and using the implicit Associations test III. Meta-analysis of predictive validity. *Journal of Personality and Social Psychology, 97*, 17–41.

Milgram, S., Mann, L., & Harter, S. (1965). The lost letter technique of social research. *Public Opinion Quarterly, 29*, 437–438.

ROY F. BAUMEISTER, Florida State University

Imagined and Genuine Opposition to New Ideas on Sexuality

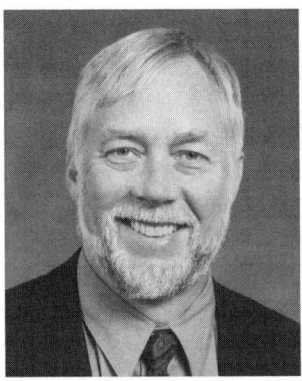

Most wise and mature psychologists counsel others to pick one line of inquiry and stay with it. The field's reward structure is set up to promote such efforts. This has never suited me. Intellectual restlessness, coupled with wide-ranging curiosity and the ambition to understand the full outlines of the human condition, pushes me to research different areas. Conceding the pragmatic difficulties of collecting data on many different topics, I hit upon the strategy of keeping my laboratory limited to a few major lines of work while conducting literature reviews of different areas. Hence, the literature review became my vehicle for exploring new realms.

I spent much of the decade of the 1990s reading and writing about what Freud told us were the two most powerful themes in human psychology, namely aggression and sex. Aggression came first, and it went reasonably smoothly. I read the vast literature on evil and violence. My conclusions were written up in a book that still remains my bestseller, as well as an article in *Psychological Review*. With the optimism of youth, I thought I had mastered the technique for doing such work.

I turned my attention to sex with the expectation that this would be another rewarding experience and that it would be all the more pleasant because of the subject matter. Researching evil and violence, after all, had required me to read all manner of unsavory and downright horrible things that people have done. I thought sex would be much more fun. I remembered the hippie slogan from my own college days: "Make love, not war." As intellectual advice, the slogan seemed to promise a chance to learn about pleasant and interesting phenomena.

The sex literature seemed at first an ideal venue for me. By all accounts, theory development was slow, and indeed many articles simply reported data with little or no theory. Partly this was due to the ongoing clash between two giant perspectives, the constructivist/feminist approach and the evolutionary approach. Mid-level theorizing had to fit one camp or the other, which meant being exposed to hostile reviewers from the other camp. Many researchers eschewed theory and simply reported their studies without much conceptual elaboration. This is precisely what a literature reviewer looks for: lots of data without overarching, integrative explanations.

Sure enough, I found patterns that seemed to have escaped the notice of previous researchers. These led to a series of literature review papers. One theme was female erotic plasticity: Social and cultural factors have a stronger influence on female than on male sexual behavior. Put another way, sexual behavior is a combination of nature and culture, but the recipe differs by gender. Male sexual behavior tends to be more natural than cultural, whereas female sexuality is the opposite (Baumeister, 2000).

Another article examined the cultural suppression of female sexuality. As a veteran literature reviewer, I was fairly certain that this would prove to be a complex and nuanced picture, full of qualifications and possibly contradictions, but to the surprise of me and my co-author, the evidence was remarkably clear and consistent. It also ran contrary to the predictions of both evolutionary and feminist theories, which for once had found an area of agreement: They both thought that men would be mainly responsible for the stifling of female sexuality. We found, in contrast, that all signs pointed to women as the main sources of influence restraining each other's sexuality (Baumeister & Twenge, 2002).

The cultural suppression paper, and some related work, led to the broadest and most integrative formulation, called sexual economics theory (Baumeister & Vohs, 2004). We knew this theory was somewhat unromantic, because it analyzes sexual interactions in marketplace terms, but the amount of information supporting it was overwhelming in quantity, diversity, and consistency. The gist is that men want sex from women and therefore give women other resources (money, respect, attention, love, commitment) in exchange for it. How much they give (the "price" of sex) fluctuates with market conditions, such as supply and demand.

These have been an engrossing set of ideas. As I said, the evidence for all of them was strong and consistent. But they have been received far less well than I had expected. Indeed, I thought that sex researchers would be more open and supportive than aggression researchers, but the opposite appears to be correct.

Another factor, I fear, is that gender is inevitably part of sexuality, and these days gender is a heavily politicized topic. Angry women and nervous men are on the lookout for any possibility that ideas might not mesh with the politically correct notions about women. (Anyone may say anything bad about men without fear of protest.)

The resistance started early. The paper on plasticity went through a review process that was about typical for that journal, but after it was accepted the editor commissioned several commentaries—by five authors, all female. They all thought I must be biased, though they contradicted each other as to what bias I had. One commentary complained that I was too biological, another that I was not biological enough. (I figured that this meant I had struck about the right balance!)

I shrugged off the assumption of bias. I really did not think that there was any value judgment in the concept of erotic plasticity. It was not obviously better or worse to be high in that trait. Yet everyone else seemed to think that bias lurked there. Later I got the impression that it is a common practice to accuse male theorists about gender of being biased.

When I was giving talks on this work, I noticed a pattern. Before the talk, my friends would anxiously or humorously suggest that I would be attacked ("crucified" was a word I heard more than once) by feminists or other radicals. Some tried to discourage me from talking about these ideas. When I asked why, they simply assumed that I would be attacked. I did not see anything in these ideas susceptible to such attacks. And, in fact, I gave plenty of talks and never once had to submit to any sort of protest or tirade. What I was saying was apparently not offensive or even controversial. Yet over and over, people assumed it would be.

This gave me insight into how ideas are sometimes suppressed. It is not always the direct stifling of an idea; rather, well-meaning colleagues and friends warn you away from ideas and even from lines of inquiry. There seemed to be the assumption that anything a man says about sex or gender will be attacked by feminists. This assumption is not without justification, though perhaps it is overstated.

I had concluded that the evidence for the gender difference in plasticity was overwhelmingly solid—but the explanation for that difference remained a mystery. One hypothesis I raised was differential strength of sexual motivation. When I raised that possibility, however, reviewers objected. They thought it quaint, unwarranted, and possibly offensive to suggest that men desire sex more than women. This led me to conduct another literature review on that topic. On this, I had a feminist co-author who started out believing that there was no gender difference in sex drive, as she told me later. But she was a scientist first and feminist second, and the data changed her mind. We found that pretty much every measure and every study pointed to higher sex drive in men. This paper, however, was not well received. The *Journal of Sex Research*, which I had thought of as a scientific outlet, dismissed it out of hand. As far as I could tell, the editor and/or reviewers had not read beyond the third page. When I protested to the main editor—the author of a leading sex textbook that speculated that women actually had higher sex drive than men—he stood by his editor and said our paper was not publishable.

I submitted the work to the annual conference of the Society for the Scientific Study of Sex. Personally, it seems hard to imagine anything more appropriate to a scientific conference on sex than a large literature review on gender differences in sex drive. They actually turned it down. To this day, I believe this is almost the only time I have ever had a conference presentation rejected.

I got the picture. Sex researchers did not want to hear this. I submitted the paper to a basic social psychology journal, where it was published, and indeed it has quickly become one of that journal's most heavily cited papers (Baumeister, Catanese, & Vohs, 2001). Yet the refusal of the sex research field even to entertain the idea still saddens and surprises me.

Similar things continued to happen with the other papers. When our review on the cultural suppression of female sexuality was about to be published, the *APA Monitor* called to interview us about it, in preparation for a featured story and possible press release. They called back with more questions and did the fact-checking, which is usually the final step. Mysteriously, this was dropped at the last minute. Our repeated inquiries as to what happened never received any response. Someone may have thought that this might go against the entrenched feminist ideas of political correctness and quashed the story, along with all coverage. There were a few similar incidents.

By now I knew not to bother with the sex journals themselves. Our paper on sexual economics went back to a leading social psychology journal, where it received extremely thoughtful and positive reviews and was soon published. Yet the field of sex research has studiously ignored it.

What did I learn from all this? I have mostly stopped research and writing about sexuality. When my graduate students do come up with some cool data on sexual behavior, we write carefully so as to placate any ideologically minded reviewers, and we avoid the sex journals. Ironically, students still seem to find their way to those papers, and each year the applications to our graduate program contain some ambitious and idealistic students who want to work with me studying sexuality. With regret, I advise them not to make sexuality the centerpiece of their research, if they want to have a fair chance at a successful research career. I tell them to specialize in relationships or interpersonal processes or something else, to build their vita around something other than sex, and to look upon sex research as a risky side venture that may be interesting—but cannot be relied on for a solid career trajectory.

The saddest aspect, however, was not the hostility and resistance from ideological antagonists; rather, it was the well-intentioned complicity of friends and colleagues who kept advising me not to study these questions, not to write or speak about them, not to risk an open-minded look at data. The work on erotic plasticity said nothing prescriptive or demeaning about women. Yet friends warned me away from it, without any specific reason. They simply thought that I would end up being attacked and suffering for it. Perhaps it is often true that ideas and lines of inquiry are stifled less because of the hostile opponents but because of the subtle, even well-intentioned pressures from friends.

As this book was being finalized, I have another book in press called *Is There Anything Good about Men?* As the title implies, it looks for some balance in understanding gender without depicting men as inferior copies of women or as evil oppressors. It has already seen some of the same issues: Well-meaning friends advised me not to write it, even though it built solidly on my previous works on culture and belongingness. I am quite sure that you would have to search long and hard to find any book on gender by a woman that is as careful to be fair and respectful to men as my book is to women. Yet we shall see whether it gets a fair hearing. I am not betting on that!

REFERENCES

Baumeister, R. F. (2000). Gender differences in erotic plasticity: The female sex drive as socially flexible and responsive. *Psychological Bulletin, 126*, 347–374.

Baumeister, R. F. (2010). *Is there anything good about men? How culture thrives by exploiting men.* New York: Oxford University Press.

Baumeister, R. F., Catanese, K. R., & Vohs, K. D. (2001). Is there a gender difference in strength of sex drive? Theoretical views, conceptual distinctions, and a review of relevant evidence. *Personality and Social Psychology Review, 5*, 242–273.

Baumeister, R. F., & Twenge, J. M. (2002). Cultural suppression of female sexuality. *Review of General Psychology, 6*, 166–203.

Baumeister, R. F., & Vohs, K. D. (2004). Sexual economics: Sex as female resource for social exchange in heterosexual interactions. *Personality and Social Psychology Review, 8*, 339–363.

NORMAN MILLER, University of Southern California, and
BARRY E. COLLINS, UCLA

A New Method for Theory Testing in Social Psychology: The Case of Dissonance

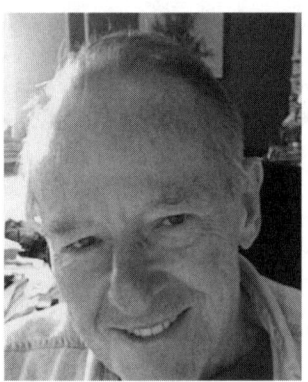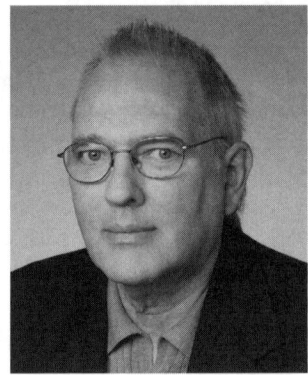

Theory testing is central to psychological science in general and social psychology in particular. Almost all theory testing in social psychology is constrained to a *critical experiment* methodology. Key variables that test an important proposition relevant to the theory are experimentally manipulated. Typically the validity of the entire theory rests on the confirmation of that one hypothesis, often in a 2×2 experiment. Sometimes, researchers can select an independent variable for which two distinct theoretical accounts make opposing predictions. For example, Festinger and Carlsmith confirmed the dissonance theory hypothesis that low justification—$1, by comparison with a $20 payment for stating that a boring task was interesting—would result in more attitude change. The Hovland learning-theory–based hypothesis made the opposite prediction. From this critical experiment approach to theory testing, the theory of the Hovland school dies and dissonance theory survives.

The moral compass that guided our own choice of research designs was formed by our internalization of the prescriptions for scientific inquiry provided by

Donald T. Campbell, our mentor. Don's compass has led us to search for (and even invent) less traveled methodological roads. Don, for example, struck out on such a new path when he made the case for unobtrusive measures as a complement to the heavy reliance on self-report, questionnaire data in 1960s social psychology. From our Campbellian, multi-method perspective, two or three variable factorial experiments are an unsatisfying basis for toppling an entire, elaborate theory that makes many predictions not sampled in the critical experiment. Moreover, the degree to which such obtained findings can be viewed as generalizable effects is limited. Critical experiments lack strong external validity because they are constrained to the particular experimental instantiations of the key theoretical variables that were manipulated, the particular context or cover story used, the particular measures used to assess the dependent variables of conceptual interest, as well as the particular sample of participants.

Structural equation modeling (SEM) approaches to theory testing provide opportunity for more elaborate and comprehensive tests of theory in that they allow simultaneous examination of a much broader array of variables than the two or three independent variables that are practical in factorial experimental designs. Especially when applied with multiple time-lagged measurement waves, SEM can approach the kind of causal analysis that forms the strength of experimental tests. Nonetheless, like any experimental test, the generalizations of the answers provided by such correlational SEM approaches are similarly constrained. As is true of every method, they too are limited to the particular measures used to operationalize key constructs and the particular respondents that are sampled.

For over 20 years we have attempted to overcome some of these limitations on comprehensive theory testing by expanding classic meta-analysis methodologies in a *theory testing meta-analytic synthesis* approach. This meta-analytic synthesis combines classic meta-analytic methodologies with a *judged variables methodology* that generates estimates of the levels of key mediating and moderating variables—variables that, more often than not, were never systematically explored in prior tests of the relevant theory and variables that are almost never measured consistently across the studies subjected to meta-analysis. This procedure adds information on numerous additional variables that can be combined with the variables manipulated or measured in studies comprising the meta-analytic database. We would like to think Don Campbell would have been thrilled by our foray into uncharted methodological ground. We think he would have approved not only because our theory testing meta-analytic synthesis approach is *different,* but also because it far more strongly invokes a *heterogeneity of irrelevances* (many measures with maximally divergent methodologies) than does the critical factorial experiment approach and thereby augments external validity.

We developed an "outside the box" methodology to obtain such bootstrapped information about specific affects and cognitions that might conceivably be antecedents mediating the link between independent and dependant variables. For this purpose judges read the method sections of the studies comprising the relevant literature and make estimates of the degree to which study participants were likely to have experienced each. In implementing this methodology, for each newly proposed mediator, judges rated its level across all the studies in the meta-analytic data set and then proceeded to the next proposed mediator. (Sometimes these judgments were made for only a key experimental condition and other times for the control condition as well.) Typically, for each judge we randomly ordered both the studies and the proposed mediators. It is important to emphasize that our purpose in such research is not to estimate a mean effect size, but instead to examine correlationally the links between the judged variables that were selected as potential new mediators and the variation in dependent measure effect sizes across the studies making up the meta-analytic database. When such links become established, note that they reflect lawfulness across variation in judges' ratings, in source of participant, and in the instantiations of independent, mediating, and dependent variables—thereby increasing external validity by exponentially augmenting the heterogeneity of irrelevancies. Finally, we note that although our obtained results cannot establish causation, one cannot have causation without correlation.

The senior author published the first exemplar of this methodology over two decades ago (Carlson & Miller, 1987). That first theory testing meta-analytic synthesis focused on theories that attempted to explain the relation between negative mood inductions and helping behavior (although in some instances, for the models that were examined, the term *hypothesis* is a more appropriate term than *theory*). Initially, this work was met with outright rejection by *Journal of Personality and Social Psychology*. It met a similar reaction at *Psychological Bulletin*, but eventually was accepted there. The most striking feature of this work was its disconfirmation of the richest and most well-developed theoretical account at the time—Cialdini's negative state relief model. A key postulate of this model was that sadness was the critical emotional state that underlies the observed relation between negative mood inductions and increased helping. Our analyses showed instead that guilt and perceived responsibility were the critical mediators, not sadness. In response to Cialdini's published criticism of our work, we reported in a second *Psychological Bulletin* article 17 additional tests of his model, all based on our original data set. None provided any support for the negative state relief model, and some presented outcomes opposite to those predicted by it. Since then we have published over ten articles that have used this theory testing meta-analytic synthesis methodology to examine a broad array of other social psychological phenomena, including such diverse topics as aggression (Marcus-Newhall, Pedersen, Carlson, & Miller, 2000), experimentally induced stress and cortisol/immune responses (Denson, Spanovic, & Miller, 2009), crossed categorization (Urban & Miller, 1998) and alcohol effects (Ito, Miller, & Pollock, 1996).

A major criticism of our approach has focused on the validity of the judges' ratings, which form a key component of our theory testing meta-analytic synthesis methodology. As previously indicated, judges (as external observers) generate estimates of the cognitive and affective states that were likely to have been induced by the experimental manipulations used in the primary research. This criticism, we suspect, was fueled in large part by the now-classic research by Nisbett and Wilson on people's inability to accurately assess why they think, feel, and behave as they do. Note, however, that our judges estimate not how they themselves would feel or think, but instead, the feelings and thoughts that the experimental manipulations were likely to have elicited in others—namely, the original experimental participants. Strikingly, in over 25 instances, our judges' ratings of study participants' emotional or cognitive states, based on their reading of method sections, have evidenced theoretically predicted construct validity. These instances have included such diverse affective and cognitive states as anticipation, anxiety, anger, brooding, challenge, cognitive overload, embarrassment, fear of losing social approval, frustration, global negative affect, guilt, happiness, importance, inhibitory response conflict, intensity of emotion, interpersonal similarity, irritation, novelty, objective self-awareness, personalization, responsibility, sadness, self-focus, submissiveness, surprise, threat, and uncontrolled repetitive thoughts. Moreover, in some of this research there is evidence of discriminative construct validity for judges' ratings of closely related emotional states, such as the negative mood states of sadness and guilt; self-focus and objective self-awareness; anxiety and objective self-awareness; and among the self-conscious emotions, guilt and shame. Numerous other researchers also have provided evidence that supports the construct validity of judges' ratings of affect and cognition.

Beyond this, we have meta-analytically confirmed the convergent validity of (a) judges' ratings of study participants' affect and cognition and (b) self-report data collected as manipulation checks in the original studies. In one article, judges' ratings were positively and reliably correlated with manipulation-check effect sizes for each of two types of experimental inductions of affect and for their judgments of each of two experimentally manipulated cognitions (Miller, Lee, & Carlson, 1991). In other work we have similarly obtained positive convergent validity correlations between judges' ratings and manipulation-check effect sizes of positive affect, sadness, frustration, negative affect, and arousal.

We are now poised to discuss the major point of this article: an attempt by the present authors to test dissonance theory by applying this theory testing meta-analytic synthesis methodology to the major paradigms that were developed as tests of dissonance theory (Kenworthy, Miller, Collins, Read, & Pollock, 2009). Relationships among multiple variables generated by the external, third-party judges (e.g., judgments about the amount of discomfort that would appear to be induced by the high and low dissonance levels of the independent variable) were examined. In previous applications of theory testing meta-analytic synthesis, we had relied on correlational, partial correlation, and regression analyses. In our application of it to dissonance theory, however, we applied structural equation analyses (SEM) to examine the shared and unique contributions of the judged variables to the prediction of dissonance effect sizes. These SEM analyses were performed within and across five key dissonance research paradigms: induced compliance, insufficient justification, disconfirmed expectancies, selective exposure, and free choice. We tested multiple models that corresponded to each of the major versions of cognitive dissonance theory: Festinger's original theory; a modified Festingerian model; Aronson's "threat to self" model of dissonance theory; and a model focusing on consequences of the dissonance-inducing act as initially developed by Collins and Hoyt, and subsequently promoted by Cooper and Fazio.

The judged variables examined in the SEM analyses were importance of the dissonance event; potential for negative evaluation; difficulty of minimizing own consequences; general psychological discomfort; guilt; embarrassment; objective self-awareness; external attribution; internal attribution; strength of experimental induction of dissonance; responsibility for others' consequences; publicness of activities; foreseeability of consequences; expectancy violations; difficulty of minimizing others' consequences; and aversiveness of own consequences.

Our results, as seen in multiple SEM analyses, showed that none of these models supported Festinger's notion that the unique variance of the variable *discomfort* mediates dissonance effects. Although discomfort was correlated with effect sizes, there was no effect of discomfort, controlling for guilt. Consistent with a conceptualization of guilt as the drive component of dissonance theory, guilt strongly predicted dissonance effect sizes, virtually irrespective of which SEM model was tested. A *post hoc* theory that integrated the role of guilt with pre-existing dissonance theories is stronger than any of the pre-existing theories in isolation.

The reviewers selected to evaluate this work for publication in *Psychological Review* and *Personality and Social Psychology Review,* along with the respective editors, unanimously and vociferously rejected our article. Most prominent among the reviewers' reasons for rejection was their contention that our judges' ratings lacked usefulness for our purpose. Given that our analyses showed that the judged variables were in fact correlated with independently obtained effect sizes, we were surprised by these reactions. What better demonstration of "validity" could there be beyond a correlation with effect sizes across the studies analyzed in this meta-analytic synthesis of dissonance experiments? Further, the patterns of correlations among the judged variables were consistent with theoretical expectation. Neither of these sets of results would appear among noisy, irrelevant variables. Given in addition the rather substantial evidence for their convergent, construct, and discriminative construct validity that we presented within the article, we found this puzzling, perhaps even bizarre.

We were also criticized for not having included shame as a judged variable. It is true that our guilt variable might be a proxy for another variable we did not measure. But this is obviously true for every social psychological study. And literally every published dissonance experiment similarly can be criticized for not having manipulated and measured additional variables. Moreover, this shortfall of all individual experiments constitutes the fundamental basis for applying our theory testing meta-analytic synthesis methodology. Finally, with respect to our failure to have obtained judgments of shame, it still remains that whatever the latent variable underlying the guilt judgments, that latent variable does a better job of predicting effect sizes than does classical dissonance discomfort.

Although we could similarly challenge other less major points raised by the reviewers, a few of their comments did lead to revisions that improved the article. Nonetheless, by and large, we have been dumbfounded by their reactions to our application of theory testing meta-analytic synthesis methodology to our tests of the several major iterations of dissonance theory. Of course it is surely typical that authors are unimpressed with the reviews that lead to a rejection of their manuscript, and this universal bias is one explanation of our reactions to the reviewers' reasoning. In this instance, however, we only wish that their reviews were critiques of a *Psychological Inquiry* target article; as hinted at in our preceding discussion, never in our careers has the opportunity to respond to reviewer comments been more inviting.[1]

Additional explanations, however, lie in implicit and explicit implications of Campbellian philosophy of science. The typical reviewer is a socially central member of the relevant subsection of social psychology, and, to use a Campbell metaphor, has internalized the norms of that *tribe*. Research that conforms to the norms of an outgroup often violates basic ingroup tribal norms; thus, they appear as heresy and generate an automatic, gut-level negative reaction. Outgroups are seen as morally inferior.

For Kuhn, science takes earthly form as a social community. The authors of this volume, along with their norms and friendship/interaction patterns, form a meta-community that operationalizes social psychological science. Psychological social psychology, however, can be further subdivided into interconnected "tribes" composed of academic "disciples." For example, Leon Festinger is the prophet of the dissonance theory tribe. The bonds that bind this particular tribal group together include (a) frequently used methodologies (e.g., the 2×2, high-impact, experimental laboratory methodology, the common use of single-item dependent measures, and a reliance on univariate statistics); (b) classic, defining empirical results (e.g., Brehm's post-decisional divergence in the evaluation of chosen and unchosen alternatives described in *A Theory of Cognitive Dissonance* and Festinger and Carlsmith's enhanced attitude change with low incentive/external justification); and (c) a large set of shared beliefs (e.g., dissonance is a drive; judged variables are invalid—perhaps a communal self-protective response to the external threat posed by Bem's self-perception theory; and situational explanations alleviate dissonance). As with most of psychology's tribes there is some consensus about favorite research questions, and there are patterns of frequent interaction (e.g., most-likely journal reviewers for their work, most-likely handbook chapter authors/book editors, friendship networks, and informal groupings at conventions).

The Harold Kelley attribution theory tribe shares a pencil-and-paper, scenario methodology (largely an anathema within the dissonance tribe). The attribution tribe also shares the belief that attribution is a cognitive, affect-free process and the belief, shared with the dissonance tribe, that the availability of a situational explanation (which results in an external attribution) is an important theoretical variable.

Consistent with dissonance tribe norms, single-item dependant variables and uni-variate statistics are common in the attribution literature.

Don Campbell's tribe is a smaller and a less tightly integrated group. Members include the present authors and the chapter authors in *Knowing and Validating: A Tribute to Donald T. Campbell* (Brewer & Collins, 1981). Although frequently misunderstood by those in other tribes, Campbellian epistemology does *not* expect an *exact replication of outcomes across methodologies*. That is the main conceptual point of Campbell's multi-trait, multi-method matrix. Some findings can be attributed to reality and some to the method being used to measure it. Thus, when a new methodology fails to replicate classic findings, Campbellians are not surprised; they in fact expect such failures to replicate. Following the multi-method norm of the Campbell tribe often requires that members invent new methods when the extant literature relies on a simple or single method. Campbell's book *Unobtrusive Measures* is a methodological innovation designed to supplement the dominant pencil-and-paper methodology of social psychology. Quasi-experimental designs are further methodological innovations to complement the extant laboratory methodology.

In conclusion, when members of social psychology tribes (other than those in the Campbellian tribe) first encounter theory testing meta-analytic synthesis, they experience it as a new methodology. Thus, it will inevitably violate their methodological norms. As a new method, it will sometimes fail to replicate phenomena that are at the core of their tribal belief systems. These norm-violating properties provide one possible explanation for the automatic negative reviewer reactions to our tests of dissonance theory. More likely than not, for some of the ingroup dissonance tribe reviewers, their negative reactions to the outgroup's (our own) work are automatic processes that are not consciously available. The reviewers' reactions to our unpalatable conclusions can be read as: "I know—intuitively—that the study is fundamentally flawed; now I have to construct justifications to support that judgment."

The strength of science, as compared with other approaches to knowledge development, lies in its ability to build on a cumulative past. Yet, as seen herein, such progress is certainly slowed by the fact that its inherent pressures toward maintaining the status quo are strong indeed.

NOTE

1. We had also submitted our manuscript to *Psychological Inquiry* but it was rejected, without review, as being unsuitable for the journal. The editor saw it as not reflecting theory that stemmed from our own prior accumulated work on dissonance theory.

REFERENCES

Brewer, M. B., & Collins, B. E. (Eds.) (1981). *Knowing and validating: A tribute to Donald T. Campbell.* San Francisco: Jossey-Bass.

Carlson, M., & Miller, N. (1987). Explanation of the relation between negative mood and helping. *Psychological Bulletin, 102*(1), 91–108.

Denson, T. F., Spanovic, M., & Miller, N. (2009). Cognitive appraisals and emotions predict cortisol and immune responses: A meta-analysis of acute laboratory social stressors and emotion inductions. *Psychological Bulletin, 135*(6), 854–858.

Ito, T., Miller, N., & Pollock, V.E. (1996). Alcohol and aggression: A meta-analysis of the moderating effects of inhibitory cues, triggering events, and self-focused attention. *Psychological Bulletin, 120*, 60–82.

Kenworthy, J. B., Miller, N., Collins, B. E., Read, S. J., Pollock, V. E. (2009). *Meta-analytic review of cognitive dissonance.* Unpublished manuscript, University of Texas at Arlington.

Marcus-Newhall, A., Pedersen, W. C., Carlson, M., & Miller, N. (2000). Displaced aggression is alive and well: A meta-analytic review. *Journal of Personality and Social Psychology, 78*, 670–689.

Miller, N., Lee, J. Y., & Carlson, M. (1991). The validity of inferential judgments when used in theory testing meta-analysis. *Personality and Social Psychology Bulletin, 17*, 335–343.

Urban, L. M., & Miller, N. (1998). A theoretical analysis of crossed categorization effects: A meta-analysis. *Journal of Personality and Social Psychology, 74*, 894–908.

NORBERT L. KERR, Michigan State University

HARK! A Herald Sings...But Who's Listening?

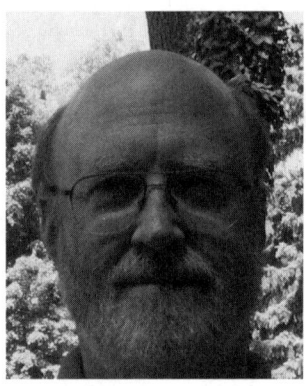

A reader quick, keen, and leery
Did wonder, ponder, and query
When results clean and tight
Fit predictions just right
If the data preceded the theory.

This little limerick, authored by a publicity-shy colleague, appears as a preface (and, I suppose, a summary) of what feels to me like my most underappreciated paper (Kerr, 1998). Such feelings, of course, are determined by two independent sources—objective signs of appreciation (e.g., where the work is published, how often it is cited, is it widely discussed, does it make it to textbooks, etc.) and one's subjective hopes for how the work will be received. The larger the gap between hoped-for appreciation and actual appreciation, the more underappreciated one sees the work (and the more disappointed one is). To harken back to this particular project, I now wonder whether my disappointment stems more from my unrealistic hopes than from any real lack of appreciation of my work. So my story, perhaps like many in this volume, may reveal as much about me as it does about the work.

A LITTLE EARLY HISTORY

It is often hard to pin down exactly where ideas come from. But I think this work had two origins—in some teaching and in some editorial work. I occasionally teach a graduate research methods course, and on one occasion I used Judd et al.'s (1991) excellent textbook. I especially liked the fact that the text pays some serious attention to topics that often get short shrift in social psychological training—for example, non-experimental methods, data coding, how to write up one's work. The latter topic is the special focus of Chapter 19, by Daryl Bem (1991), a revision of an earlier chapter (Bem, 1987). Both chapters are full of very good advice on how to write a clear, engaging, and publishable research report. But there was one piece of advice that bothered me:

> There are two possible articles you can write: (1) the article you planned to write when you designed your study or (2) the article that makes the most sense now that you have seen the results. They are rarely the same, and the correct answer is (2) ... the best journal articles are informed by the actual empirical findings from the opening sentence. (Bem, 1987; p. 172)

This text seemed to legitimize taking a genuinely *post hoc* hypothesis, one not foreseen or credited when the study was conceived and designed, and presenting it in the introduction of one's write-up as if it were a genuine *a priori* hypothesis, one that justified and guided the research. Eventually I came to call this practice HARKing (an acronym for *Hypothesizing After the Results are Known*). In fairness, Bem does not quite advocate HARKing. However, as I discussed his advice with colleagues, I found that several mentioned Bem's chapter as a justification for HARKing.

Why did this bother me so much? Initially, it was simply what looked to me like HARKing's patent dishonesty. Surely it couldn't be ethical to rewrite the true history of one's research so that one's final best understanding masqueraded as one's original understanding! However, I couldn't find any prohibition (or even mention) of HARKing in ethical guidebooks (e.g., the *APA Manual*). So, for a while, I simply contented myself with grousing about HARKing when we discussed report writing in my classes.

The other impetus for doing more than such grousing came from my experience as an associate editor at *JPSP-IRGP* in the late 1980s. While doing the editorial work, I noticed several things:

1. Authors who weren't prescient—those who presented hypotheses in the introductions to their papers that failed to be confirmed—rarely got positive reviews.
2. Non-prescient authors who presented quite reasonable *post hoc* interpretations of their findings routinely got one (sometimes both) of two types of reviews: (a) this paper is not publishable unless/until the author does another study

to independently confirm his/her *post hoc* hypothesis or (b) a revision of the paper in which the author HARKs—viz., replaces the introduction's original, inadequate hypotheses with the author's *post hoc* hypothesis—might well be publishable.

3. I kept seeing circumstantial evidence of HARKing, including (a) theoretical assumptions that didn't seem connected to the paper's central theoretical argument but that (so conveniently) helped explain some twist of the data and (b) experimental designs that failed to include conditions or measures that— given the ability of the author—one would have expected *if* an ostensible *a priori* hypothesis actually did guide the design of the experiment.

Informally discussing this with colleagues and brother/sister editors suggested that I wasn't imagining things—many others had (informally) noticed similar patterns.

EXPLORING HARKING

Gradually I moved from fretting and grousing about HARKing to studying it in somewhat more systematic fashions. I did a survey of social scientists from three disciplines to get some descriptive data (e.g., Does HARKing occur? How much? Why?) and some prescriptive information (i.e., Should HARKing occur?). The survey suggested that HARKing was widespread but that (at least some) forms of HARKing were widely seen as improper. That got me even more interested—surely it would be important to examine a practice where we might be "preaching one thing and practicing another." I started poking around for relevant prior work. My experience has been that the better the research question, the more interesting and relevant stuff you can find, but only *if* you look; confirming that many smart and thoughtful people have wrestled with the same problem can reassure you that you're working on a really good (i.e., complex, challenging, important) problem. For HARKing, I found lots of interesting and relevant stuff, scattered all over the place (in philosophy [e.g., Horwich, 1982], in cognitive psychology [e.g., Simon, 1955], in ethics, in discussions of good storytelling and writing, in statistics, in literature [e.g., Sherlock Holmes had strong opinions on HARKing]). This fed my conviction that understanding the roots and effects of HARKing was a really good problem. So did the reactions I got in my initial attempts to present my ideas to my colleagues in the early 1990s. The reactions were usually strong, ranging from outrage that I was airing "dirty linen" in a way that might damage the discipline of social psychology to outrage that anybody might ever engage in HARKing to relief that finally somebody was talking about a dilemma that authors constantly face. I seemed to be hitting a nerve.

All of this came to a head when I took a sabbatical in the spring of 1995 at Leiden University. I went alone (I was in the midst of a painful divorce [is there any other kind?]) with a head full of jumbled ideas, a suitcase full of notes, the outline of my HARKing lecture, and a vague intent to finally pull something coherent together.

Although it was a miserable time personally (e.g., intermittent long-distance calls to my four-year-old son), it was professionally an ideal sabbatical—with smart and generous colleagues (at Leiden and the many other places I peddled my traveling HARKing show), time to think and write, and an interesting problem to work on. I came back with a first draft of what would eventually become the Kerr (1998) paper.

I won't try here to summarize fully the content of the paper. Basically, I tried to clarify what might constitute an act of HARKing, summarize the results of my survey research, identify some of the forces (both psychological and professional) that encourage HARKing, identify what some of the costs of HARKing might be for science, and (reflecting my personal conviction that the costs exceed any benefits) I proposed a few ways that HARKing might be deterred. The paper was considerably improved by the encouragement and suggestions of the action editor at *PSPR*, Marilynn Brewer, as well as of many others (Pat Laughlin's comments were especially helpful).

APPRECIATED?

As I suggested earlier, by most of the objective and usual criteria, this paper is a poor candidate for being "most underappreciated." It was published in an excellent journal. It has been cited respectably (including in a couple of subsequently published research methods textbooks, the origin of my interest). A few colleagues have told me that they now require or recommend that their own research methods students read the paper. Most gratifying were the comments of several well-respected colleagues who said very nice things to me about the paper. Still, I remain deeply disappointed in the paper's (lack of) impact. Its last sentence reads, "If this article helps encourage discussion, debate, and research on HARKing, it will have fulfilled its purpose" (p. 216). But if there has been lively discussion and debate on this issue in (or outside of) social psychology since the paper's appearance, it has escaped my notice. And, as best I can tell from my perspectives as a reader, reviewer, and editor, the symptoms of HARKing in published social psychology are at least as commonplace today as when I first began my grousing.[1]

Now, it could well be that HARKing is really not a significant problem; I may have merely convinced myself that it is. More bothersome is the possibility that HARKing really is a serious problem—one worth discussing, debating, and researching—but that I simply failed to convince others of this. Maybe other chapters in this volume will echo this theme—the biggest disappointments are felt when you have tried your best to excite others about an idea or a problem that has really excited you, but failed.

So, the roots of disappointment about reactions to one's work lie at least as much in one's own excitement about the work, one's own expectations about its likely impact, as in others' actual reactions. Maybe the HARKing piece is a source of particular disappointment to me because it did not merely address a substantive social psychological problem that only a small handful of scholars also care about. (I suppose I could have nominated any of several papers of mine focused on jury behavior, social dilemmas, or group decision making as my "most underappreciated" work, although this would be a rather difficult, "Sophie's Choice" undertaking.) But the HARKing paper was not just targeted at a few fellow specialists; it touched on a problem that most scientists must confront when they sit down to write up their work. We tend to get more excited by our ideas when we think that many others will (or at least should) be similarly excited. When they aren't, it can be quite a letdown.

The reward structure in academic life is often characterized as a "lean reinforcement schedule," meaning that one has to work very long and very hard to get one's rewards. Those rewards are sometimes explicit and tangible (like recognition, interacting with interesting people, job security) and sometimes implicit and intangible (like getting to choose one's problems and scratching the itch of curiosity). While these rewards are real, they also tend to be uncertain, intermittent, and delayed. This may be why some people enjoy their teaching as much as their research, because the rewards can be more frequent and predictable: they can be garnered every Tuesday and Thursday.

AFTERTHOUGHT

In retrospect, it was probably a bit naïve (as well as delusional) to think that a single paper would ignite a firestorm of debate and controversy. This is particularly true for a practice like HARKing, which appears to be familiar, well entrenched, bolstered both by unconscious judgmental biases (e.g., confirmation bias; hindsight bias) and explicit expert advice (e.g., Bem, 1987, 1991), professionally functional, with few influential critics in high places (e.g., editors, textbook authors). As Thomas Kuhn (1996), among others, has pointed out, rapid change in scientific practice is the exception, not the rule. A better, more hopeful metaphor for mounting a challenge to a standard practice (even a demonstrably bad practice) may be the act of planting a seed, not igniting a fire. Plants, like fires, have to be carefully tended to grow. It takes a bit of the sting out of the fate of Kerr (1998) if I think of my writing the chapter you are now reading as watering a struggling plant (and not as blowing on the embers of a dying fire). And to the next generation of social psychologists, I'd echo Jackson Browne's advice:

> Into a dancer you have grown
> From a seed somebody else has thrown
> Go on ahead and throw some seeds of your own…

NOTE

1. The appearance of Kerr (1998) did have some impact, although not quite what I had hoped for. From time to time, I've had colleagues interrupt presentations of their work to assure the audience (while looking fixedly at me) that they *really* did have some particular hypothesis in hand before doing their study. Or, colleagues have come to me to ask whether one or another instance of presenting or revising a hypothesis is or isn't HARKing. On all such occasions, I assure my colleagues that I have neither the wisdom nor desire to function as a HARKing policeman.

REFERENCES

Bem, D. J. (1987). Writing the empirical journal article. In M. Zanna & J. Darley (Eds.), *The compleat academic: A practical guide for the beginning social scientist* (pp. 171–201). New York: Random House.

Bem, D. J. (1991). Writing the research report. In C. Judd, E. Smith, & L. Kidder (Eds.), *Research methods in social relations* (6th ed., pp. 453–76). Fort Worth, TX: Holt.

Horwich, P. (1982). *Probability and evidence.* Cambridge, England: Cambridge University Press.

Kerr, N. L. (1998). HARKing (Hypothesizing After the Results are Known). *Personality and Social Psychology Review, 2,* 196–217.

Kuhn, T. (1996). *The structure of scientific revolutions.* Chicago: University of Chicago Press.

Simon, H. A. (1955). Prediction and hindsight as confirmatory science. *Philosophy of Science, 22,* 227–230.

PAULA M. NIEDENTHAL, CNRS and University of
Clermont-Ferrand

Some Things Get Better With Age

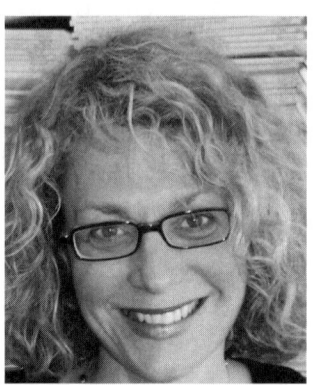

Back in the early 1980s, one of my graduate school advisors, Robert B. (Bob) Zajonc, was working on what he called the vascular theory of emotional efference (VTEE). He was very interested in the facial feedback theories, which hold that facial muscular movement can alter emotional state. But he was critical of the existing theories because he charged that they described a phenomenon without providing a full-throated, low-level mechanistic account. The VTEE advanced the radical idea that facial muscular movement could constrict venous flow by its action on the cavernous sinus. This constriction, according to the theory, would have the effect of cooling the arterial blood flow to the brain. One consequence of this cooling would be an alteration in subjective state, the feeling of emotion. Bob went on to publish some extremely clever studies in support of this controversial account (e.g., Zajonc, Murphy, & Inglehart, 1989), but not before we (Zajonc, Adelmann, Murphy, & Niedenthal, 1987) had published another paper that was based on this concern with facial expression and emotion. That paper was a 20-year roller-coaster ride and I think an important lesson in the resurrection of empirical findings.

It all started one day when Bob announced to three graduate students whom he had convened in his office that if facial expression had a causal relationship to emotional state, then the mimicry of another person's facial expression (because it produces corresponding use of facial musculature) should be a fundamental mechanism by which we know another person's emotion; one basis of empathic understanding. That sounded reasonable and cool to us, us being myself, Pamela Adelmann, and Sheila Murphy. Then Bob generated a hypothesis, typical of Bob in its wide-reaching implications: If this is so, then people who are married for a long time should grow to resemble each other. Why this is true is obvious, he claimed. People who are married are trying to understand each other's feelings all day long. If they have to mimic each other in order to really empathize, then they should use their facial muscles in a very similar way over years. Just like with any muscles, this would lead to a particular development of the many facial muscles that participate in facial expression, and because this specific development was shared by these two people, they should show increased resemblance from before the time of their wedding.

So we started the research. One of the research tasks assigned to me was the creation of the stimuli. We wanted photographs of members of married couples at approximately the time of their wedding, and also 25 years later. Through friends of my parents and other contacts I finally managed to amass photographs of 12 couples who were around 55 years old at the time of the study, and who had been married since sometime in their 20s. It was important to have separate photographs of each individual member of a couple so that other features of the photographs (such as background elements or even the brand of photographic paper) would not influence judgments of perceived similarity. Of course, since Photoshop did not exist back then, I had to reproduce the photographs so that they were about the same size and possessed the same level of contrast in the darkroom. I spent a lot of time in there. In addition to providing their photographs, we also requested each member of each couple to complete a questionnaire concerning aspects of their relationship. These data were useful because we hypothesized further that for particularly well-adjusted couples the increase in similarity over time would be even more marked.

In the primary experiment, participants saw displays of a target individual of one sex (either at the time of marriage or else 25 years later) presented above the faces of six same-aged individuals of the opposite sex over a series of trials. Of the six possible spouses, one was of course the actual spouse. In one response condition, participants were instructed to rank order the possible spouses with respect to the likelihood that they were actually married to the target individual. In a second response condition, the participants were instructed to rate the facial similarity between the target and each of the six individuals of the opposite sex. Because Bob was always trying to rule out alternative explanations before hearing about them in a nasty review, he then immediately directed us to conduct a second study in which we covered the faces of all target individuals and the six comparison stimuli with oval white masks. All that was left in each photograph was the person's hair. Then we recruited new participants to come into the laboratory and perform the same judgment tasks as the initial participants had performed. Although the idea of having participants judge which hair was likely to be the wife or the husband of the target hair may seem weird, I should say that Bob held a strong theory of participant compliance. Thus, he favored experimental instructions with no cover story: "Show them something and tell them to respond on a given scale," he said. "So what if there are no faces in these photographs. Just tell the participants to put together the real spouses." Bob figured that this second study would allow us to rule out the alternative hypothesis according to which any perceived increase in similarity of the members of married couples was due to increased similarity in the way they wore their hair, or to the fact that the lighting or photographic paper was more similar in the later photos compared to the earlier ones.

The results of the set of studies led to a clear conclusion. Compared to randomly created pairs, individuals who were married to each other grew to look more alike over the course of their marriage. Furthermore, and important for the empathy and facial feedback account, this relation was even stronger for those couples who reported that they were happy, held the same attitudes, and were basically well adjusted. The possible objection that the findings were due to similarity of features of the photos other than the faces, such as the targets' hairstyles or the grain of the photographic paper, was ruled out by the follow-up study in which the faces had been masked.

I have to say that we were very excited about these results. Bob was a great writer and he had lots of fun writing up the seemingly intuitive, but previously inexplicable, phenomenon in such a clever and scientific way. We immediately submitted the paper to the *Journal of Personality and Social Psychology*. But we didn't have to wait long for a decision letter to arrive. The editor at the time did not even send the paper out for review. In fact, I think it came back in the mail the next day. Who would have thunk it? Not us. I probably do not have to describe in detail the reaction that Bob had to the letter from *JPSP* stating that the paper was being returned without review as inappropriate. I watched him with real admiration as he stormed up and down the halls of the Research Center for Group Dynamics at the University of Michigan for most of the day. This must be an important paper, I thought then.

It was not important for science, though, as evidenced by the fact that we only succeeded in publishing it in a small, specialized journal. On the other hand, the findings had great media appeal. On August 11, 1987, the front page of the *New York Times* Science section announced that "Long-Married Couples DO Look Alike, Study Finds." We received so many requests for interviews that we started to divide them up among all of the co-authors. For example, I agreed to be interviewed by a journalist for the *Detroit News*. And I also naïvely agreed to be interviewed live on a WABC radio morning talk show in New York City. It was 6 a.m. in New York City (and in Michigan) and when I called the show, as planned, the talk show host first put me on hold. As I sat there on hold and listened to him chatting away about the early rush-hour traffic I realized that this was raw entertainment, not the news. When the host put me on the air he started out by asking me, "So, do people really look like their dogs?" I struggled and failed to have some scientific credibility. The last thing the host said was, "You know, my ex-wife is named Paula. What do you think that means about how I look?" I told him that I didn't know, and hung up, stricken. My radio interviews were over for many years.

Meanwhile, as the months went by, Bob began to receive the most mind-boggling letters from all over the world. In one, from Australia I think, a man enthused that our findings supported the idea that Eve was made from Adam's rib. A creepier letter proposed that this increased similarity was not caused by facial mimicry but rather by the fact that women absorb the semen introduced into their bodies during sexual intercourse. Such absorption, he claimed, was the cause of this increased similarity in appearance. Around the same time, cartoons and greeting cards started to appear that were premised on the idea that couples grow to look alike over the course of their marriage too. And then we really knew we had arrived when one day Bob arrived at his office and found a copy of the *National Enquirer*, an American celebrity gossip newspaper, lying on his desk. On the cover his ex-wife had written, "Turn to page 12." Page 12 featured a story whose headline proclaimed "Child Falls into Garden and is Devoured by Venus Fly Trap." Below this headline, Bob was further instructed to "Turn to page 5." On page 5 we learned that "My Baby was Born with Three Heads." Next to the surely doctored (but not by Photoshop of course) quite bizarre photograph, Bob was told to now flip to page 17, where he learned that "Couples Grow to Look Alike, University of Michigan Study Finds." The best thing about the *Enquirer* article was that it included reproductions of many photographs of American celebrity couples, such as Paul Newman and Joanne Woodward, and Pat and Shirley Boone, who had been married for a very long time and who resembled each other dramatically. I witnessed Bob give some great talks in which he showed those photos, as well as the greeting cards and the cartoons, and later I did too.

But the work had absolutely no scientific impact whatsoever. At the time they were published, no one in the social psychology community knew what to do with the findings, and so they more or less disappeared into an abyss. Then, in 2005 I was invited to give a talk at a conference held in Paris that was entitled "From Social Resonance to Agency: Multi-disciplinary Perspectives." The focus of the conference was the manner in which the brain supports facial mimicry and indeed the functions of such mimicry. My presentation was called "Who mimics whom? Constraints on imitation of emotional gesture." As an introduction to my reasoning and findings on facial mimicry at the time, I recounted the story of the old study on how couples grow to look alike over the course of their marriage. To my complete surprise, influential neurophysiologists were fascinated by the results. From their perspective these findings supported the emerging simulationist and embodied cognition accounts of how emotions are processed, and especially how empathy works. Thus, to them the findings were interpretable, exciting, and very useful.

Only several months later, I was sitting at lunch with a famous neurophysiologist who is part of the team in Parma, Italy, that discovered the mirror neuron. In a discussion of emotion and embodiment, he said to me earnestly, "I heard about a very interesting study conducted in social psychology. In it, the researchers looked at

the increases of facial resemblance of couples over the course of their marriage...."
Later that same neurophysiologist described our findings on National Public Radio in the United States, and I listened to it online with wonder. It took all those years of embarrassment, discouragement, and sometimes hilarity, but the findings were finally appreciated by scientists. I might add that my neurophysiologist friend's radio interview went rather better than my own. Trust NPR; reserve judgment for the "morning zoo" doing the traffic report.

Bob Zajonc passed away in 2008, and his passing was hard for all of those who worked with and were touched by his ideas. But one of the things he knew by that time was that those old findings had finally come back, and had come back to gain a scientific stature that they had never seen in the pages of the *National Enquirer*.

REFERENCES

Niedenthal, P. M. (May, 2005). *Who mimicks whom? Constraints on imitation of emotional gesture.* Invited paper presented at the conference "From Social Resonance to Agency: Multidisciplinary Perspectives," Paris, France.

Zajonc, R. B., Adelmann, P. K., Murphy, S. T., & Niedenthal, P. M. (1987). Convergence in the physical appearance of spouses: An implication of the vascular theory of emotional efference. *Motivation and Emotion, 11*, 335–346.

Zajonc, R. B., Murphy, S. T., & Inglehart, M. (1989). Feeling and facial efference: Implications of the vascular theory of emotion. *Psychological Review, 96*, 395–416.

JOSEPH P. FORGAS, University of New South Wales

Episodes in the Mind: Or, Beware When the Paradigm Shifts …!

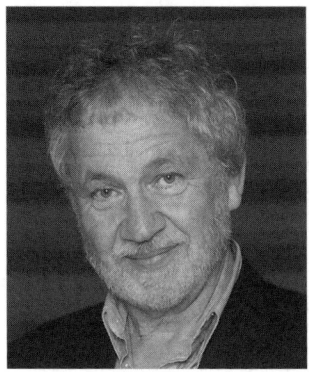

When I was invited to contribute to this fascinating volume, my first reaction was, "What a great idea!" Scientists being such an insecure species, asking them to air their frustrations and disappointments in public is likely to yield wonderful insights not only about our discipline, but also about the personalities and idiosyncrasies of us, the practitioners. To be honest, I can't wait to read about the disappointments of my esteemed colleagues. Given the highly schematic nature of most scientific communications, there really ought to be more volumes of this kind allowing us to learn from our mistakes, and to give a human face to what may often appear to the uninitiated to be a dry and highly structured enterprise.

In my case, what I consider to be my most consistently ignored or underestimated work happened rather early in my career—actually, it was my doctoral research! I feel it never received the recognition I thought it deserved. What made this even more surprising if not galling is the fact that even as a doctoral student, I was able to publish this work in the most selective journals in our field—in *JPSP, JESP,* even a chapter in the prestigious *Advances in Experimental Social Psychology* series—and I actually wrote an entire monograph summarizing the research program (Forgas, 1979, 1982). All to no avail.

So what went wrong, and why was this work so impressively ignored? And what did I learn from it? The way I see it now, my experience says a fair bit about the role of fads, fashions—you may even call them *paradigms*, if you like—in our discipline. Their ebb and flow could have a major influence on what flies and what sinks, and why.

THE ZEITGEIST

I was trained as a "proper" experimental social psychologist, and my Honours thesis dealt with group polarization and was duly published in the *European Journal of Experimental Social Psychology*. However, when I arrived at the University of Oxford to work on my DPhil, I encountered a rather strange world. It was the mid-1970s, and social psychology was officially in "crisis." The certainties of what to do and how to do it had vanished; experimentation was under attack and the paradigm was shifting under our very feet. On both sides of the Atlantic, Rom Harre and Ken Gergen thundered against laboratory experiments, Mischel's criticisms of personality psychology were just beginning to get real traction, and qualitative and interpretive methods were championed even by such giants of our field as Jerome Bruner, one of the progenitors of the social cognition movement, who was also then at Oxford.

In hindsight, the "crisis"—the rejection of the experimental method, concern with cultural and historical relativities, interest in subjective "accounts"—can be seen as a somewhat belated manifestation of some of the radical social convulsions of the 1960s. It had two major effects on social psychology: It prepared the way for the social cognitive revolution for those of us who were more empirically minded, and it gave rise to a particularly unattractive, ideologically biased, and soft-minded trend towards postmodernist discourse analysis and critical social psychology that almost destroyed empirical social psychology in the UK for the next couple of decades.

So what was a young man about to embark on a doctorate to do in such a climate? My supervisor, Michael Argyle, a kindly and supportive person, was somewhat skeptical of the radical claims seeking to demolish the empirical foundations of what, until then, appeared a reasonably successful and thriving discipline. I spent six months reading in the library, and came across a few papers using individual differences multidimensional scaling, then a fairly new technique, to analyze how people implicitly represent various social stimuli. I became intrigued by the possibility of using this method to analyze and represent the way common, everyday social episodes are mentally represented by people in their daily lives. Here was a project that could be done rigorously and empirically, yet it would yield something meaningful about the mental worlds of real people as they construe their social experiences. I was also deeply influenced by reading symbolic interactionists such as George Herbert Mead, and subscribed to the idea that an ecologically valid taxonomy of social situations and episodes was essential for the progress of social psychology.

THE WORK

The empirical work required learning quite a lot in a short time about multidimensional scaling (MDS), and adapting the technique to studying social episodes. Funnily enough, if I remember correctly it was in the Department of Forestry at Oxford that I finally found somebody who knew about MDS and was willing to explain it to me. Within a couple of years, I ran something like eight empirical studies mapping people's mental representations of the social episodes that occurred in their daily lives. Typically, participants would be asked to keep a diary for a few weeks, writing down every social episode that occurred within that period. We would then identify the most common such episodes (e.g., having lunch in college, going to a doctor, playing sport, meeting a girlfriend, etc.) and ask a second sample of participants from the same milieu to provide similarity ratings between the episodes, which would be used as the input to MDS. What resulted is a "map" or "episode space," in two, three, or four dimensions, that showed how particular individuals or particular groups implicitly represented typical social episodes in their lives.

I studied all kinds of people and groups—students, academics (including my own academic group!), housewives, rugby teams—and typically got fascinating and readily interpretable results. I was also very encouraged by early reactions to my work. My first-ever study was submitted to *JPSP* and accepted almost without revision. The second study got published in *JESP*, and in general, the reaction was encouragingly positive. I thought that I was onto a good thing with this line of research. It was solidly empirical, told us something inherently interesting and fascinating about the way people implicitly think about and mentally represent real and recurring social situations, and made a useful contribution to what even to this day is missing in social psychology: a reliable empirical taxonomy of social situations. I gave a number of talks based on this work, and the reception was universally positive.

Even before I finished my doctorate, I got a contract from a highly reputable publisher, Academic Press, to write a monograph based on my research. And during one of his visits to Oxford, Len Berkowitz also encouraged me to submit a chapter to be considered (and eventually published) in his *Advances in Experimental Social Psychology* series. So, even if my work eventually came to be ignored, it certainly wasn't for lack of any effort or success in communicating it in the best mediums of our discipline.

SO, WHAT WENT WRONG?

Well, basically, the crisis was over, and the paradigm shifted again under my feet. By the early 1980s social cognition emerged as the new way of doing social psychology. Classical social psychology focused on studying real, "impactful" behavior, albeit within the confines of rather artificial experiments. Social cognition was a partial response to what was one of the main messages to emerge from the "crisis" of the 1970s: to take more seriously what social actors think rather than just what they do, although nobody was paying any attention to affect—yet. Within a few years, rather artificial laboratory experiments were back in vogue, except instead of studying behavior, social psychologists were now studying isolated individuals sequestered in a cubicle having an interaction with a computer screen.

What was *not* happening was any renewed and enduring interest in the ecologically valid study of everyday social situations and episodes. Curiously, while the taxonomic study of personality took a great leap forward (or perhaps sideways?!) with the emergence of the Big 5 approach, the taxonomic study of social situations and episodes remained largely dormant. At any rate, my previously ever-so-promising efforts to empirically analyze people's mental representations of their everyday social episodes were not getting much attention. Citations were rather disappointing, and only a very small group of researchers such as Randy Colvin and Harry Reis maintained any interest in the ecologically valid study of social situations. Just as the generalizability of classic experiments in social psychology suffered from not having a reliable taxonomy of relevant social situations within which an experimental situation could be located, social cognitive experiments were, and still are, similarly afflicted. Except that nobody seems to mind anymore. The crisis was over, and "normal" science resumed, to use a Kuhnian phrase. My work on social episodes, even though published in the best journals, was fast sinking into oblivion.

MOVING ON

In life, as in science, so much is due to serendipity. Coincidence, luck, call it what you will, plays an important role in the way lives, careers, and scientific discoveries happen. Bill Bryson's fantastic book on science, *A Short History of Almost Everything*, which I never cease to recommend to anyone who is willing to listen, is a great testimony to this principle. In my case, after three years in my first job as an academic at the University of New South Wales, according to the generous standards of my university I was already due for six months of paid sabbatical leave. I decided to go to Stanford. Unfortunately, none of the eminent social psychologists there at the time showed the slightest interest in working with me. However, the chair of the department at the time, Gordon Bower, invited me to work with his cognitive group, who were investigating mood effects on memory and associative processes at the time.

This was a truly lucky break. Gordon has been a wonderful, generous, stimulating collaborator and friend ever since. As a result of my visit to Stanford, and the serendipitous meeting with Gordon and his research group, I started on a new research topic, investigating affective influences on social memory, judgments, inferences, and ultimately, interpersonal behavior. This time, the paradigm was right. My visit to Stanford coincided with the emergence of affect research as an important new field in social psychology, and the papers I published in this field received a far better response than did my earlier work on social episodes. The far more cheerful history of this happy collaboration has been recorded elsewhere (Forgas, 2007).

SOME CONCLUDING COMMENTS

Is there a moral to this story? Was it a mistake to do work on social episodes in the first place? Would I do it again? How does a young person know which way the wind is blowing, where the paradigm is heading, where the next big wave is coming from, the one that you can ride to success, and will not dump you in a puddle of obscurity? The short answer is, one just doesn't, and cannot know; the essential thing is to just keep on paddling. What is important is to be enthusiastic and excited about whatever you are doing, and believe in it. I am not sorry to have worked on social episodes, and one of these days I may well go back to it.

With the obvious benefit of hindsight, I think my experiences recounted here illustrate the importance of fashions, fads, and paradigms in any field of enterprise. I had the misfortune to be doing my doctoral research just at the moment when the paradigm was shifting. Unavoidably, I was influenced by what was happening in the field around me at the time. I still think today that my early work on the cognitive representation of social episodes was important and well worth doing. Interest in the empirical study of social situations, although never a "mainstream" topic, did continue to bubble along in the past 30 years. From time to time, I would be approached by researchers from all over the world with interest in my early work, I would get articles to review that dealt with related topics, and I would come across the odd paper that cited me.

And the story is not yet complete. What goes around comes around. Perhaps the time for the kind of research I did then is yet to come. Just last week, I was asked to write a promotional blurb for an excellent book arguing for a return to impactful experiments that focus on real social behavior, and calling for more attention to the real and perceived social situations in which such behavior occurs. Who knows, perhaps the paradigm may be shifting again? Stranger things have happened. The study of mental representations of social episodes may yet become of mainstream interest. If this were to happen, it would be just too bad that few researchers if any will remember and cite my early efforts on this topic.

REFERENCES

Forgas, J. P. (1979). *Social episodes: The study of interaction routines.* London and New York: Academic Press.

Forgas, J. P. (1982). Episode cognition: internal representations of interaction routines. In L. Berkowitz (Ed.), *Advances in experimental social psychology* (pp. 59–104), New York: Academic Press.

Forgas, J. P. (2007). Mood effects on memory, social judgments and social interaction. In M. A. Gluck, J. R. Anderson, & S. M. Kosslyn (Eds.), *Memory and mind: A Festschrift for Gordon H. Bower* (pp. 262–281). Hillsdale, NJ: Lawrence Erlbaum Associates.

JONATHON D. BROWN, University of Washington
Kiss My "TASS"

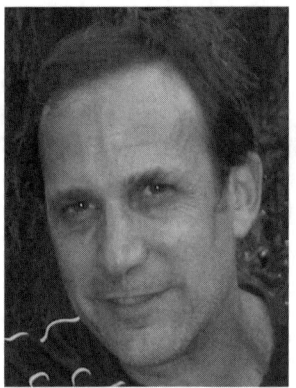

In the early 1980s, while still an undergraduate at UCLA and naïvely unaware that many social psychologists question whether personality exists, I attended a talk by Camille Wortman. During her talk, Professor Wortman admonished her audience for doubting the importance of personality processes, remarking, "If you want to believe in personality, just have two children. I did and I do."

Several years later, after my second son was born, I found myself appreciating the wisdom in Professor Wortman's remark in a particular way. As my children matured, I noticed that they differed in regard to how much discipline was needed to produce a desired behavior (or eliminate an undesired one). For one of my kids, a simple admonishment sufficed (e.g., "Don't pull the cat's fur, he'll bite you"); for the other, a great deal more was needed (e.g., "If you don't stop pulling the cat's fur I'm not going to pay for your college"). In more general terms, it seemed to me that personality often revealed itself in just this way: Individuals differ with regard to how sensitive they are to various situational pressures or stimuli. A sentimental person cries during a formulaic, romantic comedy; a competitive person plays cutthroat croquet with his nieces and nephews; and a socially anxious person feels uncomfortable during the minimum of social interactions.

I incorporated these insights into a model I called the Traits as Situational Sensitivities (TASS) model, and set about developing and testing it. It seemed to me to be a fairly obvious insight, and one that was broad and integrative. In fact, by including the terms "traits" and "situations" in the model's name, I had hoped to call attention to a basic point of intersection between personality and social psychology: To possess a trait is to possess a propensity to respond to situational stimuli in a particular way. Who could disagree?

Well, as it turned out, I was half-right. Although many people did agree, others disagreed, often vehemently. In fact, the model was met with the most polarizing feedback I've ever seen (and I've seen some polarizing feedback). Here's a sample of the feedback we received. Whereas one reviewer wrote "Hard as I try, I cannot find anything positive to say about this research," the editor who accepted our paper for publication described it as "an excellent paper that will perhaps take on a status of [an] 'instant classic.'"

In relating these comments, my point is not to disparage the peer-review process. After all, the paper was ultimately published in a top journal (Marshall & Brown, 2006), and it's too early to tell whether it will be widely cited or relegated to the "missed opportunity" heap that inspires many of the papers in this volume. Instead, I want to talk about the nature of the feedback itself. What does it say about our discipline when the same piece of research can inspire such widely divergent reactions? As I see it, two related factors bear on this question: (a) a preference for complicated, exotic arguments rather than simple, intuitive ones and (b) the inherently subjective nature of what constitutes good social psychological research.

My interest in the first of these issues began when I started working with my first mentor, Bernie Weiner. Cut from the same cloth as Fritz Heider's "commonsense" psychology, Bernie's career has been devoted to illuminating the interesting theoretical implications of everyday social interactions and perceptions. Another of my UCLA mentors, Hal Kelley, had a similar perspective. One year, Kelley and I met for lunch every week to discuss various topics of mutual interest. He ended each session by encouraging me to think carefully about the psychological richness underlying ordinary human behavior (and to do less laboratory research!).

The TASS model follows in this tradition. Its main insight is that people respond to situations differently because their personalities differ. This is by no means an earth-shattering assertion: In fact, one of the studies we reported showed that laypeople also hold this view of personality traits (Marshall & Brown, 2006, Study 2). What sets this model apart, I believe, are its implications, which are not entirely obvious. Because people react differently to situational pressures, people who are at one end of a trait distribution will be more reactive to mild forms of situational provocation than will those at the other end. However, this pattern of sensitivities will reverse when mild forms of provocation are compared with strong forms.

Marshall and Brown (2006, Study 1) illustrated this point in an experiment on aggression in response to provocation. After writing an essay, participants received either positive, moderately negative, or highly critical feedback from a fellow student.

(Of course, feedback was randomly assigned and was not really from the other student.) Afterward, they indicated how angry they were and then set a level of aversive noise the other student would (allegedly) experience during a competitive task. As the TASS model predicts, participants who scored high in hostility experienced a steep rise in anger and aggression following moderately negative feedback, but those who scored low in hostility experienced a steep rise in anger and aggression only following highly critical feedback. We have found a similar pattern of data in our research on self-esteem and emotion (Brown & Marshall, 2006) and are currently testing the model in other domains (e.g., prejudice).

The genesis of these theoretical predictions comes from everyday observations, not much different than Professor Wortman's assertion that one need only have two children to appreciate the role personality plays in shaping behavior. Unfortunately, the commonsense approach to social psychological research seems no longer in vogue. Rather than seeking to understand the ordinary and prevalent, most social psychological research focuses on the extraordinary and rare—and the more complicated the analysis and the more obfuscating the explanation, the better. Somewhere in this universe, I suspect that William of Ockham is chuckling (or cursing). Instead of following his dictum to never use complex logic when simple logic will suffice, most social psychologists have decided to never use simple logic when complex logic sounds more interesting. Of course, with the length of most articles now exceeding 30 pages, and the number of studies being reported in each paper now approaching the number of stars in the known universe, it is unlikely William is reading a lot of social psychology these days.

Admittedly, my observation is largely a matter of opinion, an admission that leads to my second point. The value of social psychological research is inherently a subjective judgment, more akin to aesthetics than science. Research areas fall in and out of fashion, and editorial decisions often revolve around which you might like better, Klee or Kandinsky, rather than the scientific merits of the research itself. Another research area of mine provides a suitable example. In recent years I have published a series of articles showing that East Asians are as self-enhancing as Americans (for a review, see Brown, 2010). But none of this research has appeared in a top APA journal. I believe this is because it runs against the current tendency to exalt cultural divergences rather than identify cultural commonalities. But why should this be? Ultimately, it is just as important to recognize cultural universals as cultural specifics, so one finding shouldn't necessarily be considered more interesting or important than another. But reviewers, editors, and readers do have a clear preference for hearing one story rather than another, and these preferences guide publication patterns.

So what would I counsel a young scientist today, as she or he begins a professional life? Here I would pass along the advice of Shelley Taylor, another of my UCLA mentors, who encouraged (and enabled) me to study the things I found most interesting, without regard to whether they were trendy or fashionable. Sure one can be pragmatic and chase grant money, but over the long haul, the best psychological research is done by those who are personally engaged in the work they do. So my advice to a new PhD is this: Open your eyes as wide as you are able, and look closely at the ordinary for the insights it reveals; follow your heart to study the questions you most want to answer; and tell people who don't like it to kiss your TASS.

REFERENCES

Brown, J. D. (2010). Across the (not so) Great Divide: Cultural similarities in self-evaluative processes. *Social and Personality Psychology Compass, 4,* 318–330.

Brown, J. D., & Marshall, M. A. (2006). The three faces of self-esteem. In M. Kernis (Ed.), *Self-esteem: Issues and answers* (pp. 4–9). New York: Psychology Press.

Marshall, M. A., & Brown, J. D. (2006). Trait aggressiveness and situational provocation. A test of the "Traits as situational sensitivities (TASS)" model. *Personality and Social Psychology Bulletin, 32,* 1100–1113.

JOHN H. HARVEY, University of Iowa

The Slow, Halting Appreciation of Close Relationships Research

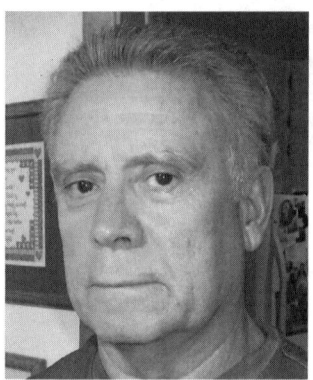

In this commentary, I will discuss my earliest experience in doing, trying to publish, and gaining research support for work on close relationships. I will link my experiences with the pioneering work on relationships of Harold Kelley, one of my mentors. But first let me backtrack to the point at which I became involved with Kelley in studying attributional and close relationships processes in the 1970s.

I had the great fortune of working on my MA and PhD with Jud Mills at Missouri in the late 1960s. He suggested I apply for an NIMH-funded postdoctoral fellowship to work on attribution theory, which he arranged with Hal Kelley at UCLA, 1971–72. This time at UCLA was a wonderful era for studying attribution, since it came soon after the UCLA conference on attribution in the 1960s (Jones et al., 1972). I am glad that there is so much on attribution and related phenomena in the present volume, including Weiner's interesting retrospective "Publish and Perish." Not only was UCLA, with Kelley and Weiner leading the way, a hotbed of attribution work, it also was producing some fine social psychology scholars in the 1970s, including the editor of this book, Bob Arkin, who took a methods class with Kelley (and me an assistant) in the early 1970s.

I will now develop the "underappreciation" part of the story. In a 1978 paper entitled "Attribution in the context of conflict and separation in close relationships," Gary Wells, Marlene Alvarez, and I compared women's and men's attributions about conflict in 36 unmarried heterosexual couples. The couples were selected because they had lived together for at least 6 months and had indicated that they were experiencing a high degree of conflict. Each member of the couple answered a 65-item attribution measure that asked them to indicate their own attribution and predict their partner's attribution of the importance of different causal factors (e.g., financial, faithfulness) in their conflict. The results showed various differences in gender (e.g., males rated incompatibility in sexual activities as more important than did females). Of greater significance, we thought, were the patterns of inaccuracy in own versus predicted importance of various causes of conflict. For example, males showed significant inaccuracy in overestimating females' attribution of importance to sexual incompatibility.

This research represented one of the earliest studies of attribution in conflict and separation in close relationships. Harold Kelley and his colleagues (Orvis et al., 1976) earlier had found in a study of 41 young couples that divergent causal attributions are prominent features of conflict situations. Our work amplified on that theme and pointed to the role of inaccuracy in understanding other's perspective. It was as if these young couples could not readily get inside the minds of their partners in evaluating the importance of certain factors in leading to their dissatisfaction and conflict. Later in the 1980s and 1990s, investigators such as Frank Fincham and Tom Bradbury refined this area of work to a considerable degree in probing how attributions are related to relationship satisfaction and stability.

Of relevance to the present volume was the experience that my colleagues and I had in trying to publish our work. Similar to the fate of Kelley and colleagues (Orvis et al., 1976), our work was rejected by the *Journal of Personality and Social Psychology*, and other major outlets at that time. The concerns focused on the small N and self-selected nature of the sample, the issue of causality, and whether the work advanced understanding beyond common sense. A similar outcome occurred in subsequent grant submissions based on this research. As the reader will see, these early papers on attributions in relationships were published in a volume edited by myself, Bill Ickes, and Bob Kidd—hardly the type of peer review response desired! But the papers, including the one by Orvis et al., were widely cited for the next two decades.

What is important, I think, for the development of the field of close relationships in psychology was Harold Kelley's efforts in developing the close relationships field in social psychology. He did not give up in the face of adversity in bringing respectability and enthusiasm to these new fields. He developed a forum among early scholars representing different domains of psychology and sociology to make the case for a science of relationships. The quest was to make this case just as tenable as the case for a science of any other type of social psychological phenomenon. Kelley unveiled these plans in a 1977 meeting at Vanderbilt University that my colleagues and I organized to honor Fritz Heider, the founder of attribution theory (more on Heider below).

As Kelley was accustomed in doing (before with attribution scholars, and at the end of his life with his work in bringing together scholars to develop an atlas of interpersonal situations), Kelley created a group to study and advance the cause of relationships research in psychology. He sought and gained the support of other early workers in studying the psychological aspects of close relationships (Ellen Berscheid, George Levinger, Ted Huston, Anne Peplau, Andy Christensen, Don Peterson, Evie McClintock, and myself) to develop a 4-year set of workshops for the group of scholars to come together, debate, analyze, synthesize, and write a major book outlining key features in the science of relationships. Kelley et al. (1983) was the product of these meetings. The meetings were generously funded by the National Science Foundation, and I think it is fair to say the resulting product had an enormous influence in stimulating work on relationships.

Now as an aside, a little bit of the story of Fritz Heider needs to be woven into this discussion. Heider would have been a superb contributor to this book. Heider essentially lived this book regarding the underappreciation of one's ideas. As alluded to in Weiner's article in this book, Heider spent over 40 years, from the time of his completion of his PhD dissertation in 1920 at the University of Graz in Austria to the 1950s, trying with little success to gain recognition for his unique theories of interpersonal and person perception and interpersonal relations (Heider, 1958). These ideas were the forerunners of attribution theory in social psychology. Before Heider died in 1988, along with my colleagues Bill Ickes and Bob Kidd I had the extraordinary opportunity to interview and spend time with him and his gracious, accomplished wife Grace Heider (both of whom had been professors at the University of Kansas) in the 1970s and 1980s. Heider described his depth of hurt in giving talks in the 1920s and 1930s and having his ideas laughed at and dismissed (Heider, 1976). Heider finally began to be given his due when Ned Jones and Hal Kelley imported his ideas to their seminal works on attribution in the 1960s. His is a classic tale of perseverance to see one's ideas received and appreciated. No less than social psychology's founder Kurt Lewin, Fritz Heider has had a theoretical influence on social psychology that is both pervasive and enduring.

As for my own later work on attribution, the research with Wells and Alvarez was a precursor to the development of an emphasis on how people develop stories ("account-making," exemplified in Harvey, Weber, & Orbuch, 1990) containing specific attributions, description, and emotional expression in trying to understand major events in their lives. Respondents in this early work pointed me and others to the possible role of contextualized attributions—as part of packaged narratives about events in their lives. Further, this interest in how people understand conflict and endings in their close relationships led to my broader interest in how people deal with major losses of all types, and to later research, writing, and teaching in the field of loss and trauma. As shown in a volume edited by Harvey and Miller (2000) and in a journal I created in 1995, *Journal of Loss and Trauma* (Taylor and Francis

Publishers), there are innumerable links among concepts such as attribution, closeness, and loss and trauma. To a very large degree, Kelley's approach to integrating perspectives, ideas, and scholars from diverse fields is reflected (albeit not nearly as well, nor grandly) in my own work as a social psychologist.

What is invaluable for young scholars to take from our experiences is the importance of tenacity in persevering to gain credence for one's work, even in the face of harsh rejection. There are many great essays in this volume that reflect the importance of "fighting the good fight" in the interests of one's passions about ideas. One has to believe in and sometimes fight for what one does and thinks is critical as a scholar and a person. I hope that Heider's story will be passed on to future generations of social psychologists as a standard for perseverance in believing in one's ideas. Kelley was a major figure in psychology when he first started receiving rejections for his relationships work. I was even discouraged from creating an undergraduate course on relationships in the mid- to late 1970s by the Vanderbilt University Arts and Sciences Dean on the ground that the field was too "soft." I thank my colleagues then at Vanderbilt, such as social psychologists Bill Smith and Don Thistlethwaite, for standing behind me in creating this course, which Ellen Berschied has referred to as probably the first offerings on close relationships in a psychology department in the United States.

In commenting on the present piece, Bob Arkin made the perceptive point that it is ironic that close relationships work is so central to social psychology today, yet back in the 1970s and 1980s, it was such a hard sell to get the field and its theories and methods accepted. He went on to note that really the hard sell was getting the "social" in social psychology accepted.

In looking at the vast domain of work on relationships today in social psychology and related fields, the inimitable vision of Hal Kelley continues to be reflected both in the melding of cross-disciplinary and international perspectives on relationships and in the ideas such as interdependence that are so integral to this field.

REFERENCES

Harvey, J. H., & Miller, E. D. (Eds.) (2000). *Loss and trauma: General and close relationship perspectives*. Philadelphia: Brunner/Mazel.

Harvey, J. H., Wells, G. L., & Alvarez, M. D. (1978). Attribution in the context of conflict and separation in close relationships. In J.H. Harvey, W. J. Ickes, & R. F. Kidd (Eds.), *New directions in attribution research* (Vol. 2, pp. 235–59). Hillsdale, NJ: Lawrence Erlbaum.

Harvey, J. H., Weber, A. L., & Orbuch, T. L. (1990). *Interpersonal accounts: A social psychological perspective*. Oxford: Basil Blackwell.

Heider, F. (1958). *The psychology of interpersonal relations*. New York: Wiley.

Heider, F. (1976). A conversation with Fritz Heider. In J. H. Harvey, W. J. Ickes, & R. F. Kidd (Eds.), *New directions in attribution research* (Vol. 1, pp. 3–18). Hillsdale, NJ: Lawrence Erlbaum.

Jones, E. E., Kanouse, D. E., Kelley, H. H., Nisbett, R. E., Valins, S., & Weiner, B. (Eds.) (1972). *Attribution: Perceiving the causes of behavior*. Morristown, NJ: General Learning Corporation.

Kelley, H. H., Berscheid, E., Christensen, A., Harvey, J. H., Huston, T., Levinger, G., McClintock, E., Peplau, A., & Peterson, D. (1983). *Close relationships*. San Francisco: Freeman.

Orvis, B. R., Kelley, H. H., & Butler, D. (1976). Attributional conflict in young couples. In J. H. Harvey, W. Ickes, & R. F. Kidd (Eds.), *New directions in attribution research* (Vol. 1, pp. 353–386). Hillsdale, NJ: Lawrence Erlbaum.

ICEK AJZEN, University of Massachusetts–Amherst

Is Attitude Research Incompatible With the Compatibility Principle?

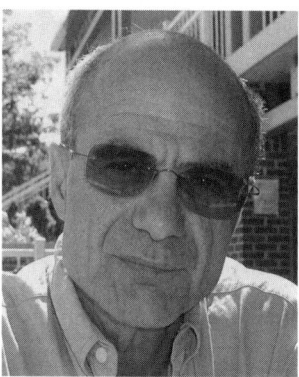

Perusing the primary journals of social psychology I am struck by the nature of contemporary research on attitudes and related constructs. In the majority of studies, attitudes, cognitions, affective reactions, and various more or less stable individual differences are treated either as dependent variables or as correlates of other such variables; in relatively few studies are these factors used to predict and explain actual or intended behavior. Thus, current research explores, among many other things, the factors that influence, or correlate with, intergroup stereotyping and prejudice, right-wing authoritarianism, social dominance orientation, moral judgments, self-esteem, implicit versus explicit attitudes, emotion regulation, and value orientations. I interpret this feature of contemporary attitude research to reflect a general consensus that attitudinal variables are essential determinants of human social behavior and that it is, therefore, important to study their antecedents and the interrelations among them.

From a historical perspective, this consensus—if it in fact exists—is most gratifying, for I remember a time when social psychologists were criticizing the attitude construct and other broad dispositions for their demonstrated inability to predict actual behavior. That attitude again occupies a central place in social psychological theorizing is, at least in part, attributable to our better understanding of the relation between attitudes and behavior. I like to think that my own theoretical contribution, such as it is, has aided in this development. Central to my efforts has been the emphasis on compatibility in the definition and assessment of attitudes and behavior. According to the principle of compatibility, attitudes predict behavior only to the extent that both are defined at the same level of generality or specificity in terms of their target, action, context, and time elements (see Ajzen, 2005, for a discussion). The low predictive validity of attitudes in early research can, I would argue, be traced largely to a lack of compatibility: Very general attitudes toward a target—without reference to action, context, or time—were used to predict specific actions performed in a particular context and at a given point in time, and sometimes directed at an incompatible target as well. Thus, investigators might assess attitudes towards Blacks in general and then assess performance of a particular behavior, such as having one's picture taken with a specific Black individual, in the context of an effort to promote interracial understanding. By way of comparison, when care is taken to maintain compatibility between attitude and behavior, correlations are generally very strong. This can be accomplished by assessing attitudes at the level of the specific behavior that is to be predicted, or by aggregating different behaviors in the domain of interest to achieve a level of generality that corresponds to the general attitude (see Ajzen, 2005).

If our introductory social psychology textbooks are an indication, the principle of compatibility is well understood and widely accepted; yet its translation into practice is less than universal. It is still common to see a great deal of incompatibility in studies that use attitude as an independent variable to predict behavior. A good case in point is research on prejudice and discrimination. A moment's reflection reveals that both prejudicial attitudes and discriminatory behavior are very general constructs. Prejudice is directed at a certain target group, be it African Americans, Hispanics, Muslims, gays, or the elderly. No particular action or context is indicated when attitudes toward such groups are assessed either by means of explicit or implicit methods. Similarly, discrimination is a broad behavioral category that generalizes across a variety of specific actions and contexts. Consider, for example, anti-Muslim discrimination. To obtain a valid, representative measure of this behavioral category, we would have to aggregate across diverse actions directed at Muslims in different contexts, such as talking, or refusing to talk, to Muslims; sharing jokes about Muslims; inviting a Muslim couple to one's home; attending a Muslim wedding; eating at a Muslim-owned restaurant; recommending a Muslim candidate for a position; and voting for a Muslim candidate for political office. According to the compatibility principle, a measure of prejudice toward Muslims should be a good predictor of the overall aggregated tendency to behave in a discriminatory manner, even though this general attitude would not be expected to predict performance of any individual behavior very well.

Of course, an investigator might well be interested in understanding the factors that influence performance of a particular behavior in relation to Muslims, say biases in hiring decisions. In that case, the principle of compatibility suggests that the investigator assess attitudes toward hiring the particular Muslim applicant, not general prejudicial attitudes toward Muslims. The particular beliefs that inform the behavior-relevant attitude may help explain biases in hiring decisions where more general attitudes toward Muslims would not.

These ideas are well understood, but their importance is largely underappreciated. Examination of research on prejudice and discrimination reveals a frequent failure to observe the principle of compatibility. On the behavioral side, common paradigms in this research involve hiring decisions in which research participants are given a job description and asked to read the résumé of an applicant for the position who is said to be either Black or White; judicial decisions involving judgments of guilt or innocence in gender- or race-related job discrimination or criminal law suits; and nonverbal behaviors, such as eye contact, physical distance, or smiling in interactions with members of a certain group. An attempt is then made to predict these specific judgments and actions from general measures of prejudice toward the group in question. Although studies of this kind can reveal interesting patterns of findings, the relations between the general prejudicial attitudes and the relatively specific behavioral criteria tend to be modest in magnitude, whether explicit or implicit attitude measures are obtained. This conclusion is confirmed by the results of 32 studies in the domain of racial attitudes and behavior included in a broader meta-analysis of the attitude–behavior relation (Greenwald, Poehlman, Uhlmann, & Banaji, 2009). The mean correlation for the prediction of discriminatory responses from explicit attitude measures was 0.12, and the mean correlation for the prediction of these responses from implicit attitude measures was 0.24. When the synthesis included data from all 122 research reports that dealt with attitudes and behaviors in a variety of different domains, the corresponding mean correlations were 0.36 and 0.27. These correlations are of about the same magnitude as those that, in the past, have led investigators to despair of the attitude construct (see Wicker, 1969).

If general attitudes are such poor predictors of narrowly defined individual behaviors performed in a particular context, why do investigators continue to examine predictive validity in this fashion? The answer, I believe, is that we are all convinced of the central importance of attitudes in our lives. It seems intuitively obvious that the way we think and feel in relation to an issue, group, or event greatly influences our decisions and actions. Consistent with Allport's (1935) definition of attitude, and empirical evidence to the contrary, we then proceed to overgeneralize this expectation by assuming that our broad attitudes have a strong effect on each and every one of our behaviors in relation to the attitude object. As social psychologists we take pride in our recognition of the importance of the situation or context as a determinant of social behavior. The principle of compatibility takes account of this insight by suggesting that either we focus on attitudes toward performing a particular behavior in a given context, or that we aggregate different behaviors and thereby generalize the context. Yet when it comes to attitude research, and especially research on the attitude–behavior relation, investigators often disregard the context, relying instead on broad dispositions to explain specific behaviors, behaviors that, by necessity, occur in a particular context. Perhaps the time has come to make sure that attitude research is compatible with the compatibility principle.

REFERENCES

Ajzen, I. (2005). *Attitudes, personality, and behavior* (2nd ed.). Maidenhead, UK: Open University Press.

Allport, G. W. (1935). Attitudes. In C. Murchison (Ed.), *Handbook of social psychology* (pp. 798–844). Worcester, MA: Clark University Press.

Greenwald, A. G., Poehlman, T. A., Uhlmann, E., & Banaji, M. R. (2009). Understanding and using the implicit association test: III. Meta-analysis of predictive validity. *Journal of Personality and Social Psychology, 97*(1), 17–41.

Wicker, A. W. (1969). Attitudes versus actions: The relationship of verbal and overt behavioral responses to attitude objects. *Journal of Social Issues, 25*(4), 41–78.

DAVID A. KENNY, University of Connecticut

Change We Cannot Believe In

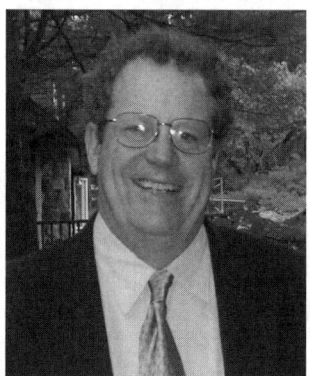

It is never good to start a paper with an apology, but I am going to do so anyway. In a book by social psychologists mainly talking about social psychology, I am going to discuss methodology. At the end of the paper, I return to social psychology.

My first solo-authored article in an APA journal was a paper on how to measure the effect of an intervention in a non-randomized study when you have a pre-measure. The title of the paper was "A quasi-experimental approach to assessing treatment effects in the non–equivalent control group design" (Kenny, 1975). According to Google Scholar, the paper has about 164 citations, and so the paper has had some impact. However, today, the paper is almost never cited. Why do I think this paper has merit (beyond the mere fact that I wrote it!)?

Let me start with some background. Consider a study of weight loss with a pre–intervention measure of weight, called here a *pretest*. Some people receive an intervention and the others serve as a control group. However, assignment to conditions is not done randomly. This design was called, by Campbell and Stanley (1963) in their classic work, the non–equivalent control group design. Due to nonrandom assignment, when we look at the pretest, we would likely see that the groups differ (e.g., in this case, the treated units weigh more than the control units). How do we control for or adjust out this pretest difference?

One idea, often labeled as naïve (by those who do not like the idea!), is to compute a change or gain score: Take the posttest minus the pretest and use that difference score as the outcome measure. Sometimes we do this without even realizing it. For instance, in most studies of blood pressure, we routinely just subtract the baseline or pretest score. Other times, we conduct a repeated measures analysis of variance, where time (pretest vs. posttest) is the repeated measure. I will refer to this approach as "change scores."

The other idea is to "covary out" the pretest. In the 1970s, we used the analysis of covariance, but today we would use the general linear model. We estimate a regression equation for the posttest, and we use treatment (i.e., a dummy variable: 1 = treated and 0 = control) to predict the posttest and we also include in that regression equation the pretest. There is an old-fashioned approach called "residualized change scores," which can be equivalent to covarying out the pretest. I will refer this approach as "covarying out."

There are two very different approaches to this problem, and these two different approaches can give very different answers. The fact that they give different answers has been called Lord's paradox (Lord, 1967). Which of these two methods is right? Methodologists take sides with most, though not all, lining up on the "covarying out" side. As the statistician Donald Rubin said to me once, "Why would you not want to weight the pretest in a way that maximally explains the posttest?" Some very intelligent people (e.g., Holland & Rubin, 1983) have argued that the two approaches answer different questions, but I think that misses the issue. The question we want answered is the following: If we want to remove the effect due to non-random assignment (what Campbell and Stanley [1963] called *selection*) to measure a treatment effect, do we covary out the pretest or use change scores? What is the answer to this question?

The answer I give in my 1975 paper is, "it depends." There are situations where change scores are right and there are situations where "covarying out" can be right. The key idea in the 1975 paper is that we need to think about the pretest in terms of components. I argued that the pretest has three theoretical components. The first is a part that does not change over time. The paper focused on that part of the pretest that is due to the population in which the person is a member. I should have referred to this part as a *trait*, and did so in subsequent work (Kenny & Zautra, 2001). Basically, this component, labeled G in the paper, does not change over time. The second part, labeled Z in the paper, changes over time. Finally, there is a third part, labeled E, that is essentially random with respect to time, and we often refer to this component as a measurement error. What I was saying is that you could break up all the causes of the pretest into three parts: a part that does not change, a part that changes some, and a part that completely changes (i.e., is random over time).

We now ask the question: Which of these components determines selection into treatment groups? That is, which of these different components of the pretest is correlated with the treatment? If it is the unchanging component that determines selection, then change scores are justifiable if we can assume that the component is also present in the posttest to the same degree. When we compute a change score, we subtract off a biasing term that is equally present in both the pretest and the posttest.

If, however, selection is based on the entire score, then you need to covary out the pretest. That is, the logic of "covarying out" is that selection is based on the score itself. While this can be plausible in some instances (what Campbell and Stanley [1963] call the regression discontinuity design), normally errors of measurement do not figure into selection. We can use the pretest as a covariate, but we need to make some sort of correction for measurement error in the pretest.[1]

The paper then provides a very general framework to help researchers decide whether to use change scores or to covary out the pretest. I will admit the paper has problems and limitations (viewing trait differences solely in terms of group differences and over-emphasizing measures of standardized change), but I think that it provides a framework for resolving Lord's paradox.

Part of the lack of acceptance of the article is due to the fact that most methodologists and statisticians seem to hate change scores. If we think about it, change scores are not so naïve after all. When we are trying to understand an outcome variable and we have a variable that we need to adjust for or control, we can either add the variable to the equation on the right side or we can add the variable to the left side by redefining the outcome variable. We adjust on the right side by adding the variable we want to control as a covariate, and adjust on the left side by transforming the variable itself.

Let me give a simple example. Suppose that we are looking at the effect of altitude on murders and we use elevation to predict the number of murders in 100 United States cities. Obviously, we need to control for population size. Could we not control for population by entering in as a variable and "covarying out" its effect? That is, we put population on the right side of the equation. But that is not what we should do. Rather, we should put population on the left side of the equation: We take murders and divide by the city's population.

In essence, the debate over change scores and covarying is a left side versus right side debate. When we covary out the variable, we put it on the right side, and when we compute a change score we put it on the left side. It is not inherently better to put the variable on the right side of the equation!

So what does this have to do with social psychology? My 1975 article sounded a very general theme that has cut across both my methodological and substantive work. That theme is that variables that we measure are not what they appear to be, but, rather, lurking behind them are multiple, hidden variables. As has been discussed here, this is the key point of the 1975 paper: Lurking inside of the pretest are three components. I have also examined social perception in the same way (Kenny, 1994). Consider the social perception that Sam sees Mary as intelligent; I believe that perception reflects many hidden variables:

- How people see others in general
- How Sam sees people in general

- How Mary is seen in general
- How Sam particularly sees Mary

I feel that we can understand person perception only if we break that perception up into components. I get the feeling that many of the people who read my work see that I can find interesting things when I break social perception into components, but they never buy into the idea that components are meaningful. They see them as some sort of statistical fiction. I see them as real. In fact, as a student of Donald T. Campbell, I believe what we observe is fallible and very misleading, and observations are mere shadows of true unobserved realities awaiting discovery.

We can view these components, whether of pretests or social perceptions, in terms of different levels of analysis. For instance, the trait component in a measure is at the level of the person, whereas the error is at the level time within person. Within social perception, there are the levels of person (both perceiver and target), relationship, and group. Thus, my obsession with components is really an obsession with the idea that what we observe reflects multiple levels of analysis. It is gratifying to begin to see that many other social scientists are accepting such a multilevel perspective.

Finally, another central idea contained in the 1975 paper is the idea of factorial invariance, another idea of Donald T. Campbell. When we measure the pretest and posttest, we might want to consider that components have an equal effect on both. If the assumption of factorial invariance is plausible, there is much that we can learn in our analyses of longitudinal data.

NOTE

1. The paper also discusses a key consideration that is almost never discussed today: the timing of selection. Even if you have selection based on the entire score, if the time point at which selection takes place is at a point halfway between the pretest and posttest, change scores would often provide a better way to control for selection than does covarying out the pretest.

REFERENCES

Campbell, D. T., & Stanley, J. C. (1963). Experimental and quasi-experimental designs for research on teaching. In N. L. Gage (Ed.), *Handbook of research on teaching* (pp. 171–246). Chicago: Rand-McNally.

Holland, P. W., & Rubin, D. B. (1983). On Lord's paradox. In H. Wainer & S. Messick (Eds.), *Principles of modern psychological measurement: A festschrift for Frederic M. Lord* (pp. 3–26). Hillsdale, NJ: Erlbaum.

Kenny, D. A. (1975). A quasi-experimental approach to assessing treatment effects in the non-equivalent control group design. *Psychological Bulletin, 82*, 345–362.

Kenny, D. A. (1994). *Interpersonal perception: A social relations analysis.* New York: Guilford.

Kenny, D. A., & Zautra, A. (2001). Trait-state models for longitudinal data. In A. Sayer & L. M. Collins (Eds.), *New methods for the analysis of change* (pp. 243–63). Washington, DC: American Psychological Association.

Lord, F. M. (1967). A paradox in the interpretation of group comparisons. *Psychological Bulletin, 68*, 304–305.

RAMADHAR SINGH, Indian Institute of Management
Bangalore, India

Imputing Values to Missing
Information in Social Judgment

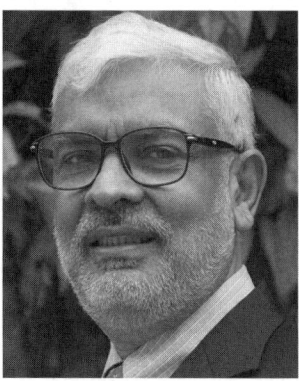

In the early 1970s, I was fascinated by information integration theory. According to Norman H. Anderson (1971), people assign values to different pieces of information about a stimulus and integrate them according to the *adding, multiplying,* or *averaging* rule in their overall judgment of it. Thus, judgment involves a chain of processes of *valuation, integration,* and *response production.* Valuation translates the physical stimulus into its psychological value and weight. The former represents its location along the dimension of judgment; the latter indicates its importance in the overall judgment. Integration unitizes not only the value and weight of one piece of information but also those of other pieces of information available for judgment. Psychologists reported considerable evidence for the pervasiveness of cognitive algebra in human judgment.

One method of distinguishing the adding rule from the averaging rule for two pieces of information in any judgment was to cross the levels of the first factor with those of the second factor and to also include the levels of each factor separately, typically in a repeated-measurement design. For example, desirability of romantic partners can be a sum or an average of the information about their attractiveness and temperament. If judgments of desirability are taken from information about their attractiveness and temperament presented together as well as separately, then the adding and averaging processes can be identified by factorial plots of the data and test of the interaction term in analysis of variance (ANOVA).

To diagnose a rule, two steps are required. First, plot the means from the compound information and perform ANOVA. If the factorial plot of the data exhibits a pattern of parallelism, there will be only the two main effects. The pattern of parallelism would imply either an adding or averaging rule. Second, also plot the means from information presented alone and do another ANOVA. If the pattern is still parallel with only two main effects, then the rule is adding: Information about attractiveness adds to the effect of temperament information; so does temperament information add to the effect of attractiveness information.

However, if the pattern of parallelism is violated by inclusion of the means from information presented alone and the interaction effect is significant, then the rule is averaging. The rationale is simple: Averaging of attractiveness information with temperament information would dilute their respective effects. So, the slope of curves based on both attractiveness and temperament information should be shallower than the slope of the curve based on either the attractiveness or temperament information presented alone.

This phenomenon of diluted effects of information can be important. For example, should you present all your experiences in your résumé when seeking a job, or only the best information about yourself? The answer depends on whether the prospective employer would integrate the information using an adding or averaging process.

Other models of cognitive algebra are diagnosed similarly. Multiplication of the attractiveness and temperament information would produce a linear fan pattern (i.e., a greater divergence between curves at the high than low level of any factor) and an interaction effect in the ANOVA. Further, the interaction effect would reside in the Linear × Linear trend. A linear fan pattern is also possible if the rule used is averaging but lower compared to higher values of attractiveness and temperament have greater weights (Anderson, 1971). Thus, the multiplying and averaging rules are distinguishable by the slope of the curve for information presented alone. According to the multiplying rule, the curves based on any single piece of information alone should still form part of the linear fan pattern. According to the differential-weight averaging rule, however, the curves based on any single piece of information should violate the linear fan pattern.

A DIFFERENT PERSPECTIVE

In everyday life, people know something about a person and infer other attributes (e.g., motivation, ability, sincerity). Information available for these inferences is hardly complete. To make a judgment, people impute values to missing information. So, imputations are inherent in all day-to-day social cognition and raise doubt about a method that relies exclusively on responses to the information presented alone as the grounds of rule diagnosis. I did not want to disregard imputations about missing information only because they were unknown.

For making judgments of gift size, for instance, people need information about both the generosity and income of the donors (Graesser & Anderson, 1974). Information about either generosity or income is logically insufficient. If people do make judgments about gift size, it means that they imputed some value to the missing information. Consequently, I began my research in 1975 to demonstrate that people impute values to missing information, and that such imputations can be ascertained from the cognitive algebra employed.

In the initial two experiments, participants received information about annual income in Indian Rupees (Rs.) and generosity of hypothetical persons and estimated the size of gift they might have sent to a family whose house had burned down. Figure 3.1 presents the mean judgments of gift size as a function of income (listed as curve parameter) and generosity (listed on the horizontal axis). The four

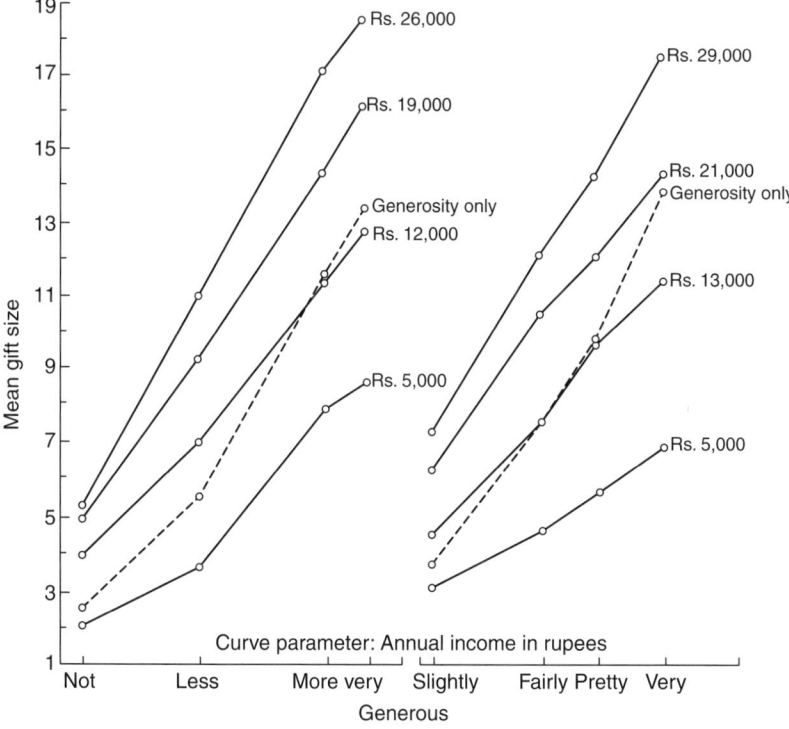

Figure 3.1.
Mean judgment of gift size as a function of income and generosity of stimulus persons. The five curves of the left panel are from the first preliminary experiment and those of the right panel are from the second preliminary experiment. The solid curves are from 4 × 4 (Income × Generosity) design identical to that of Grasser and Anderson (1974); the dashed curves are based on information about generosity information alone. Copyright © 1991 Lawrence Erlbaum Associates, Publishers. Reprinted with permission of Norman H. Anderson and Taylor and Francis Publishers.

solid curves show the judgments when information about both income and generosity was supplied. They form a linear fan pattern as if the multiplicative rule were operative (Graesser & Anderson, 1974).

To distinguish between the averaging and multiplying rules, I added another condition, represented by the dashed curves in Figure 3.1, which corresponds to judgments from information about generosity alone. In each experiment, the generosity-only dashed curve crosses over the second solid curve. This crossover violated the linear fan pattern and hence raised doubts about the multiplying rule (Graesser & Anderson, 1974), but argued for a differential-weighted averaging rule (Anderson, 1971).

An averaging interpretation had to ignore the possibility that participants might have made imputations about the missing income information. I considered two possible patterns of imputations. One is imputing a single-fixed value, presumably around the average of the specified values in the experiments. If so, the generosity-only curve is essentially the same as the other conditions and the dashed curve should form part of the linear fan pattern according to both the multiplying and averaging rules. With this pattern of imputation, however, neither rule could explain the results of Figure 3.1.

Imputations might also depend upon the value of the given information. An ungenerous person might be expected to have lower income than a generous person. In this case, the dashed curve should cross over one of the solid curves, as is indeed evident in Figure 3.1. According to this second pattern of imputation, the inferred value of income increased as generosity increased on the horizontal axis. With such a pattern of imputation, both rules can explain the results of Figure 3.1.

Given these results and interpretations, I felt convinced that the widely popular crossover test cannot always distinguish the adding rule from the averaging rule or the multiplying rule from the averaging rule if imputations were allowed. However, if the integration rule itself is established in some other ways, the two patterns of imputations about the missing generosity or income information can be confirmed.

RESEARCH PROGRAM

During the next seven years, I conducted six new experiments. Experiments 1 to 3 were intended to (a) rule out the possibility that a nonlinear use of the response measure might also produce a linear fan pattern, and (b) confirm the second pattern of imputation from the generosity information given. Toward these goals, I crossed multiple pieces of information about generosity with a single piece of information about income and also took judgments from one of those pieces of generosity information presented alone. Three results were consistent. First, the effects of multiple pieces of generosity information on judged gift size had the pattern of parallelism, which supported the conclusion that the given response measure was used in a linear, instead of nonlinear, way. Second, the Income × Generosity effect had the linear fan pattern, as if a multiplying rule were operative. Finally, the imputed value of missing income increased with the increasing value of the generosity information given.

In Experiments 4 and 5, I studied imputations about missing generosity or income information. Again, the rule seemed to be multiplicative; the missing generosity information was imputed a fixed value; and the imputed value to the missing income information increased with the increasing value of the generosity information given.

In Experiment 6, I studied the multiplying rule by manipulating the value and reliability of the generosity and income information. This method avoided the problem of imputation and exclusively tested the rule itself. Reliability of information should affect its weight. So, the multiplying and averaging rules made sharply contradictory predictions. According to the former, an increase in the reliability of generosity information should amplify the effect of the income information and vice versa. According to the latter, however, an increase in the reliability of generosity information should decrease the effect of the income information and vice versa. Results supported the prediction of the multiplying rule and rejected the prediction of the averaging rule.

Findings advanced the literature in two ways. First, the cognitive algebra for judgment of gift size was indeed Gift size = Generosity × Income. Second, the rule *per se* should be used to diagnose the patterns of imputations about missing information. Methodologically, therefore, the focus shifted from diagnosing the rule from responses to missing information to determining imputations about missing information from the rule used.

DISSEMINATION

I made my research public in a working paper of the Indian Institute of Management, Ahmedabad, India, in 1984. At the invitation of Norman H. Anderson, I submitted the report as a chapter in his *Contributions to Information Integration Theory, Vol. II: Social*. Seven years later, the book was published (Singh, 1991). In his preface to my chapter, Anderson noted:

> This chapter . . . is a tour de force in cognitive psychology. One problem concerns imputations, that is, inferences about missing information. A second concerns an alternative interpretation of the ostensible multiplying rule, Gift size = Generosity × Income. . . . . Singh solves both problems with thorough precision. . . . . This conjunction of theory and experiment represents a new standard of excellence. (p. 142)

The working paper itself was cited by a few colleagues in journal articles and in chapters of some books during the late 1980s. Anderson himself cited the published chapter a few times in some of his own later writings. So, what I considered an important contribution to social psychology has remained heretofore underappreciated!

UNDERAPPRECIATION

To me, this work seems to have remained underappreciated for three reasons. One is the choice of publication outlet. This research could have been submitted to the *Journal of Experimental Psychology: General* as I had originally planned instead of as an invited chapter in Anderson's (1991) volume. Another is the decline in the popularity of information integration theory since the mid-1980s. Still another reason could be the somewhat hard-to-grasp methodology. Both the precautions during experimentation (e.g., anchors, fillers, practice session) and complex analyses (e.g., breaking down of the effect into trend components, individual analyses) made the work less engaging to social psychologists at large.

The importance of the phenomenon of imputing information in social psychology still seems underappreciated. However, Irwin P. Levin and his colleagues explored the fascinating and entirely common imputation of quality of a consumer product from its price, a phenomenon of critical importance in marketing. Still more generally, most psychological experiments present some kind of information or experience in a restricted setting, and the results are usually interpreted without considering that people may read more into the information than the experimenters intended (i.e., participants are likely to impute information well beyond what they are given). Being mindful of the prospect of such imputations could inform the direction of many psychological research programs.

On a personal level, my respect for psychology as a science and my subsequent research were very much based on the rigor and sophistication in hypothesis testing that information integration theory provided me with during this experimental work. The demonstration that imputations about missing information, based on the information given in social judgment, was a truly enjoyable puzzle to solve for me and a contribution that still seems to have widespread application!

ACKNOWLEDGMENTS

I thank Nazar Akrami, Colleen F. Moore, Joseph J. P. Simons, and Melvin J. Yap for their comments on previous versions.

REFERENCES

Anderson, N. H. (1971). Integration theory and attitude change. *Psychological Review, 78,* 171–206.

Graesser, C. C., & Anderson, N. H. (1974). Cognitive algebra of the equation: Gift size = Generosity × Income. *Journal of Experimental Psychology, 103,* 692–699.

Singh, R. (1991). Two problems in cognitive algebra: Imputations and averaging versus multiplying. In N. H. Anderson (Ed.), *Contributions to information integration theory, Volume II: Social* (pp. 143–180). Hillsdale, NJ: Erlbaum.

PART IV

Phenomena and Findings

SUSAN T. FISKE, Princeton University

Whatever Happened to Schema-Triggered Affect?

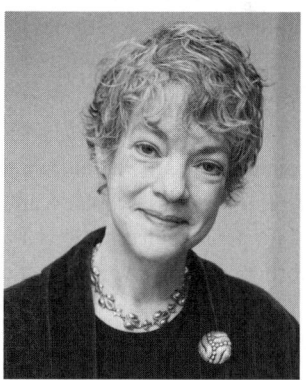

Upon hearing that someone else had just published the study they were planning to do, Jud Mills reportedly told his collaborator that he was glad, because now they did not have to do that study. Since hearing this story, I have (mostly) taken a less paranoid attitude to being scooped. This, of course, is easier once tenured.

My very own first new idea as a fresh PhD was to swim upstream against the cognitive tide sweeping social psychology, to make a case for affect. The first wave of social cognition research focused on social knowledge structures (self schemas, personality prototypes, social categories), all exciting at the time, but a little cold. My hunch: Social expectations invariably import affective baggage. Schema-triggered affect was born (Fiske, 1982). The theory was simple. Categorization not only cues cognitive associations, but also triggers affective responses. Schema-triggered affect, what's more, relied on instant categorization, not on memory for the data that originally generated the affective tag. As obvious as this may seem in retrospect, at the time it was a bizarre idea, that schema match determines affective responses.

My little lab had a great time designing schema-triggered-affect studies, some on close relationships, others on political person perception, and still others on stereotyping. The first, on old flames, asked female undergraduates, in the guise of a multi-part study, to complete a personality checklist for themselves, a same-sex best friend, and a past or current romantic partner. After a filler task rating the personalities of two videotaped conversationalists, participants began the alleged third part of the study, rating people they were about to meet. As an alleged control, they first rated facial photographs for their similarity to "the kind of guy you have been attracted to in the past." Participants then received a personally tailored stimulus person, who did or did not resemble their old flame on traits and appearance; they rated him on several positive emotions and several negative ones. Full matches (i.e., on both personality and appearance) elicited the most positive and the least negative emotions, as well as being preferred for a social group, rather than a work or discussion group. Complete non-matches elicited the least positive affect, and the lowest preference for all three groups.

So far, so good. But the partial matches showed confusing intermediate patterns, and when reviewers were rightly dubious about the lack of controls for sheer positivity, we caved to self-doubt. Besides, Susan Andersen subsequently conducted a wonderful program of research on transference, way more rigorous, scholarly, and convincing than anything we had done. She would get people's description of a significant other, feed it back to them disguised as another person, and measure the similarity of their reactions to the significant other and the doppelganger. One of her critical controls was yoking people to someone else's significant other, which then eliminated the valence issue as an alternative explanation (for a theoretical culmination, see Andersen & Chen, 2002).

We also tried to apply schema-triggered affect to political candidates and to outgroups, a common object in traditional attitude research. Our empirical work there also was promising but spotty. One study targeted the then-major presidential contenders (it was this long ago: incumbent Carter, candidates Reagan, Bush, Brown, Kennedy; we all know how that ended). Participants read the same "intimate campaign portrait," but applied to one of the five candidates. The insider description portrayed the candidate as what we had pretested to match undergraduates' prototype for a smarmy politician: slick, ambitious, vain, and fickle. Not surprisingly, this politician, whichever of the five candidates he allegedly was, generated much negative affect and scant positive. However—and this was the crucial comparison— this portrait was reversed and turned into an anti-politician (honest, selfless, etc.), rather a saint. When applied to each of the five candidates, feelings ran positive instead of negative, and Democrats quite intended to vote for him. When the prototype described a neutral, ordinary person (nebbish), affects ran neutral, and Republicans preferred him. Matching candidates to the smarmy politician stereotype disqualified them for both parties' voters.

To remedy the obvious confound (more negative traits in the politician portrait than the anti-politician one), another study applied a mixed, ambiguous politician/

anti-politician portrait to photos that stereotypically resembled politicians or not, according to pretesting. So we manipulated visual fit but held the traits constant and open to interpretation. We also assessed participants' political expertise (according to a standardized knowledge test). Experts apparently acknowledged the stereotypic politico face, if he was labeled a politician, and their negative schema-triggered affect condemned the stereotypic pol, but not if he had a nonstereotypic face or a different label (person, executive). For political novices, this schema-matching effect did not appear. Again, these studies were not flawless, and we caved before obstacles and objections.

Our final scientific foray into schema-triggered affect capitalized on campus stereotypes of engineers ("vegetables") versus artists ("fruits"), and gay versus macho guys. This study finally unconfounded content and schematic match by using each stereotype's content for the discrepant match to its yoked partner (that is, an artist who behaves like an engineer, or vice versa, is discrepant, but the same overall valence remains if the same behaviors are schema-consistent for one label and switch to be schema-consistent for the other). Indeed, collapsed over particular stereotypes and their content, these negative stereotypes elicited lower evaluations when matched than when discrepant. Thus schema-match determined affect, even holding information constant across conditions.

A later version of this study did appear (Fiske, Neuberg, Beattie, & Milberg, 1987), so these studies laid the groundwork for the continuum model of impression formation (Fiske & Neuberg, 1990). And quite honestly, in these early efforts, I was swimming against the tide without a guide or a life preserver. I simply did not appreciate the importance of relentlessly persevering on a good idea, calibrating methods, fine-tuning analyses, until we had it right. I also regret not getting publications for my stalwart research assistants during that learning curve, but a Google search suggests that they are doing quite well for themselves despite my flaws as an early mentor.

Besides, a splendid research program was simultaneously showing that attitude objects trigger evaluation upon immediate appraisal (for an overview, see Fazio, 2001), which seemed to me to make the schema-triggered affect point far better than anything we had done. And other brilliant research has shown that even subliminal priming of categories can have breathtaking effects on affect and behavior (e.g., Bargh & Williams, 2006).

My lab's other lines of research from this period eventually took priority, as did the Social Cognition (1984) text, but nostalgically, I wish we had possessed the self-confidence, the wit, and perhaps that life preserver to have kept swimming. Still, we can't really complain about being underappreciated: The original chapter proposing schema-triggered affect (Fiske, 1982) ranks a surprising 7th among my most-cited publications, and another chapter updating the fine points of schema-triggered affect (Fiske & Pavelchak, 1986) ranks 11th in citations of my work. And who can complain, when other people did both the theory and the research much better than we did or would have done? The field

has appreciated and absorbed those people's remarkable insights, to the benefit of all concerned. And now we don't have to do those studies.

REFERENCES

Andersen, S. M., & Chen, S. (2002). The relational self: An interpersonal social-cognitive theory. *Psychological Review, 109,* 619–645.

Bargh, J. A., & Williams, E. L. (2006). The automaticity of social life. *Current Directions in Psychological Science, 15,* 1–4.

Fazio, R. H. (2001). On the automatic activation of associated evaluations: An overview. *Cognition and Emotion, 15,* 115–141.

Fiske, S. T. (1982). Schema-triggered affect: Applications to social perception. In M. S. Clark & S. T. Fiske (Eds.), *Affect and cognition: The 17th annual Carnegie symposium on cognition* (pp. 55–78). Hillsdale, NJ: Erlbaum.

Fiske, S. T., & Neuberg, S. L. (1990). A continuum model of impression formation, from category-based to individuating processes: Influence of information and motivation on attention and interpretation. In M. P. Zanna (Ed.), *Advances in experimental social psychology* (Vol. 23, pp. 1–74). New York: Academic Press.

Fiske, S. T., Neuberg, S. L., Beattie, A. E., & Milberg, S. J. (1987). Category-based and attribute-based reactions to others: Some informational conditions of stereotyping and individuating processes. *Journal of Experimental Social Psychology, 23,* 399–427.

Fiske, S. T., & Pavelchak, M. A. (1986). Category-based versus piecemeal-based affective responses: Developments in schema-triggered affect. In R. M. Sorrentino & E. T. Higgins (Eds.), *Handbook of motivation and cognition: Foundations of social behavior* (pp. 167–203). New York: Guilford Press.

E. TORY HIGGINS, Columbia University

Priming Creative Behavior: Priming *How* Things Work Rather Than *What* Things Are

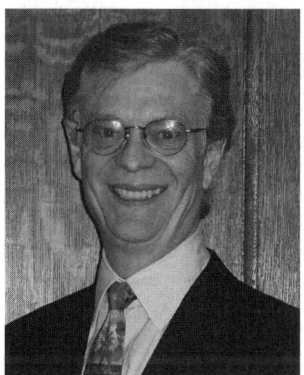

Let me begin with the original title of my "underappreciated" article, which in 1980 appeared in *Journal of Experimental Social Psychology* (Higgins & Chaires, 1980): "Accessibility of interrelational constructs: Implications for stimulus encoding and creativity." The readership of this journal was (and still is) mostly social psychologists. Now take a look again at the title of the article. Is there a single word that suggests something about social behavior? Is there a single word that was a "hot-button issue" for social psychologists in 1980? So what was I thinking? How did this happen?

Well, I don't really know what I was thinking, but I do know what happened. In late 1979, I received a telephone call from Bob Wyer. Bob was the editor of *JESP* at the time. A couple of years earlier, he had accepted for publication in *JESP* another paper with the title, "Category accessibility and impression formation" (Higgins, Rholes, & Jones, 1977)—what became known as the "Donald" study. Like the Higgins and Chaires (1980) paper, this paper had the then-unfamiliar "accessibility" word in the title. However, and critically I believe, it also had the very familiar phrase "impression formation" in the title, and in 1980 impression formation was a major issue in the person perception literature (which itself was a relatively hot area in social psychology).

Bob was finishing his term as editor and he telephoned me to ask whether I had anything new in my research program on "accessibility" that I could submit before the end of his term. I told him that I had nothing relevant for *social* psychologists. Undaunted, he asked me if I had anything relevant for *psychologists*. I said that I had some work that had just been rejected by *Science* for being too specialized for the general readership of that journal. I told Bob that it was strictly a cognitive psychology paper. He said that was "fine" because social psychologists could benefit from learning more about basic cognitive mechanisms. He said that he could not promise the paper would be accepted, but he could promise that the review process would be quick. This was early in my career. I was untenured. "Quick" sounded very good to me! So I sent him my paper with William (Bill) Chaires, which was Bill's Senior Thesis at Princeton University. Within just a few weeks, I heard back from Bob with his usual exhaustive comments—and, fortunately, they were suggestions for a "revise/resubmit" rather than a rejection. I resubmitted several weeks later, and again in just a few weeks, received back a shorter list of Wyer suggestions (down to just a few pages). I responded in a few weeks and received an acceptance a week later. The paper appeared a few months later. The entire process from initial phone call to final printed article was less than 7 *months*! To this day, it is my personal record—thanks to Bob Wyer!

As the saying goes, that was the good news. The bad news was that the paper never had the impact that I expected it would. Or that Bob expected it would. Indeed, Bob still tells me that he believes that it is my best paper. And I have heard that as well from a small handful of other social psychologists. It is time now to describe what exactly was the work that myself and a few others believe has been underappreciated—although in this case "ignored" would be a more accurate characterization than "underappreciated"; only a handful of people ever read the paper.

PRIMING AND CREATIVE BEHAVIOR: THE "DUNCKER CANDLE PROBLEM" STUDIES

From 1968 to 1972, I had worked with Janellen Huttenlocher on verbal reasoning problems. When I went to Princeton in 1972, I became interested in problem solving more generally. I became especially fascinated with "creativity" problems in which people must break set or functional fixedness in order to see things differently. One way that things can be seen differently is to represent them in a different way. My earlier work on accessibility (Higgins et al., 1977) had shown that recent priming could determine how input information was later categorized. Specifically, this earlier research demonstrated that activation of a stored category through exposure to a category-related word in one situation could determine how an ambiguous behavioral description was later categorized in a separate situation. For example, prior exposure to either the word "stubborn" or the word "persistent" as part of one study can cause participants in a later unrelated study to characterize a target person's ambiguous "persistent/stubborn" behavior as being either stubborn or persistent, respectively. And this accessibility effect occurs without people being aware that the priming influenced their judgment. Could such a temporary increase in a construct's accessibility from recent priming also facilitate creative insight?

This apparently straightforward extension of my earlier work on priming and accessibility was actually not so straightforward. To appreciate why this is the case, I need to describe the actual research that was conducted. The creative insight problem that Bill Chaires and I selected in 1976 was Duncker's (1945) famous *candle problem*:

> Subjects are seated at a table on which there is a cardboard wall, a candle, a full book of matches, and a box filled with thumbtacks. Subjects are told that their task is to affix the candle to the cardboard wall so that the candle burns properly but does not drip wax on the table. The difficult part of the problem is to think of using the box as a platform for the candle, rather than just as a container for the tacks. The critical factor in solving the problem appears to be how subjects encode the box filled with thumbtacks.

Thanks to my Princeton colleague at the time, Sam Glucksberg, we knew that the difficulty of this problem derives from the fact that most people naturally think of the box as *just a container* for the tacks—as a "box of tacks." For individuals to solve the problem, they need to change set, *un*fix the function as container, and think of the box instead as something that an object can be *on* rather than as something that an object can be *in*; i.e., think of the box as a potential platform for the candle! It is the smallest thing that is the problem here—the relational construct "of." The problem with the "box *of* tacks" representation of the stimulus is the relational construct "of." The relational construct "of" associates the box with the tacks in a relational manner in which the box and the tacks are a united whole. This highlights the box's function as a container of the tacks rather than as a *separate* object that can have a function that is independent from the tacks, such as functioning as a platform for another object.

How might the stimulus of the box filled with tacks be represented in order to separate the box from the tacks? The answer is to represent the stimulus instead as a "box *and* tacks." This should differentiate the box from the tacks, which would establish the box as an independent object. This, in turn, should make the problem easier to solve because the box as an independent object can more easily be recognized as a potential platform for the candle. If this were the case, then the trick would be to somehow prime the "and" construction, making "and" temporarily more accessible than "of" for representing the stimulus in the candle problem. Importantly, rather than priming "platform" versus "container" as semantic constructs like those primed in previous psychological studies, it would be just the relational constructs "and" versus "of" that would be primed. *It would involve priming a function rather than a content.* This was in 1976; this kind of priming effect had never been tried before.

The next question was how to carry out such priming. Taking our clue from the earlier Higgins et al. (1977) priming and accessibility study, we accomplished this by again separating the priming situation from the categorization situation (i.e., the "unrelated studies" paradigm). When the participants arrived, we told them that we were studying the effects of interference on long-term memory. They were told that they would be shown a series of photographed objects to remember, and that those participants in the "interference" condition would have to work on another task before recalling the objects. In fact, all of the participants were in the "interference" condition, and the "interference" task was the Duncker candle problem.

The "objects to be remembered" were various common objects, such as a banana, a football, a scissors, and so on. In addition to these stimuli that are normally designated by a single word, there were other stimuli involving a container with its contents that are normally designated by a phrase, such as a bowl containing cereal and a carton containing eggs. The experimenter labeled what appeared on each slide, such as saying "banana" or "scissor" when these slides appeared. In the "Of" priming condition, the slides with container-content objects were labeled as "bowl *of* cereal," "carton *of* eggs," and so on. In the "And" priming condition, these same slides were labeled as "bowl *and* cereal," "carton *and* eggs," and so on.

After exposure to the same set of photographed objects, all participants were taken to a separate room where the objects of the candle problem were on a table hidden under a cloth. Ostensibly as part of the introduction to the problem, the cloth was removed and the participants in Study 1 were simply asked to write down their descriptions of the objects. Once they had written their descriptions, the study was over. The participants were extensively debriefed to determine whether they were suspicious about the true purpose of the study or saw any connection between the "memory" study and the "interference" study other than what the instructions had said about the candle problem being an inference task for the memory task. The participants did not report any suspicions or any other connection between the tasks.

Study 1 found that the participants in the "And" priming condition were much more likely than those in the "Of" priming condition to spontaneously describe the box in a manner that separated or differentiated it from the tacks, such as writing down the word "box" and the word "tacks" on separate lines, rather than writing down the phrase "box of tacks." This study demonstrated that it was possible to use priming and accessibility to influence whether the box and the tacks were later represented in a differentiated manner or not.

Now the question was whether our priming and accessibility manipulation could influence creative behavior in the candle task. If participants were *not* asked to name the objects after the cloth was removed, and only represented the objects *covertly*, would prior "And" priming in the separate "memory" task produce more creative behavior than prior "Of" priming? We addressed this question in Study 2. There was a time limit of 10 minutes to solve the problem. Study 2 found that in the "Of" priming condition, the average time working on the problem was 9 minutes and only 20% of the participants solved the problem. In contrast, in the "And" priming condition, the average time was 4.5 minutes and 80% of the participants solved the problem—a dramatic improvement in creative behavior!

These findings had significant implications. For the field of creativity, it highlighted the importance of distinguishing between the *availability* and the *accessibility* of constructs stored in long-term memory (see Higgins, 1996). Creativity is often conceptualized in terms of novel ideas being available to some individuals but not others (i.e., the "genius" vs. the rest of us). Creative insight is often described as something new, a discovery that someone makes, which suggests making some idea available that was not available before the mental breakthrough. However, we cannot prime and increase the accessibility of a stored construct that is not already available. What made this priming unusual was that it did not increase the accessibility of a specific semantic construct like "platform"; rather, it increased the accessibility of the general relational construct "and." These studies demonstrated for the first time that it is possible to prime and increase the accessibility of a *function* rather than a *content*. And the function itself, as was the case in this research, can be already available. The general relational construct "and" was already available to the participants, but it was less accessible than the alternative function that was *functionally fixed* to the stimulus (the "of" construction). Priming the "and" construction increased the accessibility of the less familiar function—it *unfixed* the stimulus— thereby facilitating creative behavior. (Why wouldn't the readership of *Science* be interested in this new perspective on what it means to be creative?)

Beyond its implications for understanding how creativity works, our studies demonstrated that priming and accessibility had a potential power over thought and behavior that was far greater than had been appreciated before. Study 2 was the first study to demonstrate that priming could influence someone's behavior on a task—and not just any behavior on any task, but creative behavior on a difficult problem-solving task. Rather than priming and accessibility being restricted to influencing people's recognition of *what things are* (e.g., someone's behavior is "persistent" vs. "stubborn"), it can also influence people's recognition of *how things work*—in this case, by differentiating the box from the tacks, the recognition that a box can function as a platform and not just as a container. Study 2 showed that we can prime general functions and not just specific contents, and this can increase insightful behavior without people being aware of the source of their insight. It provides a new tool wherever such insight is needed, from helping students at school or team members at work solve a task problem, to helping patients in clinical therapy solve a personal problem.

My personal lesson from this "underappreciated" research program is to *know your audience*. As I told Bob Wyer, this research was more central to cognitive psychology issues at the time than to social psychology issues. Thus, I should have submitted the research to a cognitive psychology journal. Indeed, it may still be the case that the readers of this volume are not the ideal audience for this chapter because the research is still more relevant to cognitive than social issues *per se*. But things have changed in social psychology and in psychology generally. Over the past 30 years, it is social psychologists who have contributed most to understanding the nature and consequences of priming and accessibility. It is social psychologists who have discovered what amazing effects priming and accessibility can have (for a recent review, see Eitam & Higgins, in press). And for an audience who appreciates these discoveries, my early research on priming *how* things work rather than *what* things are, this early demonstration of a priming effect on creative problem solving, was a forerunner to unlocking the hidden and unexpected power of priming and accessibility on human behavior. It is a power that continues to fascinate me and that I continue to try to understand (see Eitam & Higgins, in press).

REFERENCES

Eitam, B., & Higgins, E. T. (in press). Motivation in mental accessibility: Relevance Of A Representation (ROAR) as a new framework. *Social and Personality Psychology Compass*.

Higgins, E. T. (1996). Knowledge activation: Accessibility, applicability, and salience. In E. T. Higgins & A. W. Kruglanski (Eds.), *Social psychology: Handbook of basic principles* (pp. 133–168). New York: Guilford.

Higgins, E. T., & Chaires, W. M. (1980). Accessibility of interrelational constructs: Implications for stimulus encoding and creativity. *Journal of Experimental Social Psychology*, *16*, 348–361.

Higgins, E. T., Rholes, W. S. & Jones, C. R. (1977). Category accessibility and impression formation. *Journal of Experimental Social Psychology*, *13*, 141–154.

JOEL COOPER, Princeton University

What's in a Title? How a Decent Idea May Have Gone Bad

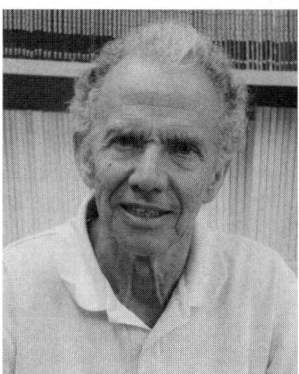

Writing about my most underappreciated idea requires a bit of hubris. It presupposes that I had an idea worthy of appreciation, that I continue to appreciate, but that fell on deaf ears. The last of the triumvirate is easy. There are many candidates from which to choose. It takes some hubris to believe that one of those ignored publications deserved more attention than it received. Nonetheless, there is one line of research that has lain dormant for a few decades and, at the risk of deluding myself, I occasionally think may be rediscovered someday.

The story goes back to my days as a graduate student at Duke University, where I worked with the outstanding scholar of interpersonal perception, Edward E. Jones. I believe that if Ned were alive today, and if he had been able to contribute to this volume, he would have chosen the same project.

ATTITUDE CHANGE AS AN INTERPERSONAL STRATEGY

Ned and I worked to meld his interest in strategic impression management with my own interest in attitude change. Naturally, the idea was more his than mine, but

I thought it was a fascinating one. Will people adopt attitudes as a strategic device to manage their impressions and, if so, when? There are some uninteresting occasions in which people may distort their attitudes to manage impressions, such as when you, as a meat-eating, plastic-bag-using consumer, find yourself in a roomful of people wearing Save the Planet buttons and carrying their canvas grocery sacks. In such a circumstance, in the idle conversation of the moment, you might like to keep your opinions to yourself. But if you must comment, you might express positions that are in line with what you think the people in the room would like to hear: your love of vegetable tofu and your disdain of ever using a plastic bag at the grocery store.

We were interested in the more subtle variations of this pressure. Imagine this scenario: Suppose you are a college student chatting with a classmate whom you knew had acted in an arrogant or unpleasant way toward one of your instructors. That instructor then enters the room and recognizes the partner. You are mortified that this respected instructor may think that you are unpleasant and arrogant, too, by dint of your association with your partner. You need to signal your independence. The instructor engages the two of you in a discussion that focuses on some of the important political issues of the day. Your colleague speaks first and you discover that you and your partner agree. Will you show your independence by changing your attitude in an unwanted direction, just to show the instructor that you are not at all like the arrogant bore? We suspected so, and we designed our most underappreciated study to show it.

Ned, having been trained in the Lewinian tradition, was not interested in scenario studies—that is, the ubiquitous reliance on asking participants to *imagine* a complex situation. In this tradition, if a participant was supposed to be in a room with an arrogant, obnoxious other, then, doggone it, there had to be a real obnoxious other in the room. And that was me.

We also reasoned that people in the strategic dilemma we designed would be in quite a conflict. They would prefer not to distort their attitudes on meaningful issues such as support for free speech and opposition to the war in Vietnam if they did not absolutely have to, but they also needed to differentiate themselves from the obnoxious other person (me). So, if the participant was in the room with the arrogant bore *and there were other discernable differences* between the participant and me, then the participant would not have to change his attitudes to demonstrate the difference. We decided to use mode of dress and region of the country as alternate ways to show differences or maintain similarities.

Ned once described the procedure of our study as a three-ring circus. Acting as the confederate, either I played the role of an obnoxious, unlikable other subject or, using my best acting skills, I acted in a likeable, friendly manner. To show my similarity with the real participant, I used regional accents to signal that we came from the same or different parts of the country. Ned was a stickler for noticing how a person dressed, so the other way we signaled similarity or dissimilarity was to change clothes to try to match as closely as possible (or not) what the participant was wearing. That required a genuine clothing wardrobe with sweaters, t-shirts, jeans, shorts, slacks, and even sports jackets. The participant arrived first and then, depending on condition, I was able to take a quick look at his appearance, change clothes, and enter the room.

With all of this going on, we actually obtained our predicted results. Compared to an attitude survey that the participants had filled out in another context, we found the attitude change we had expected. When I had been obnoxious and dressed and spoke in a manner similar to the participant, the participant expressed a different attitude than he had expressed on a confidential attitude survey. If I had been obnoxious but my dress and accent indicated that I was different from the participant, then the participant showed no change of attitude. If I had been like-able, then participants were more than pleased to have the same attitude as I did, regardless of my mode of dress or my regional accent. The results showed that people were motivated to express deviance from an unlikable other, even at the expense of expressing attitudinal positions with which they formerly disagreed—such as opposing civil rights legislation, supporting tuition increases, and squashing students' rights to protest.

WHAT IS IN A TITLE?

Ned had uncannily good judgment about whether a paper would be accepted for publication in *JPSP*, and when this three-ring circus of a procedure turned into real results, he was confident this study would see the light of day. Therefore, I was too. There was the question of what to call the paper. I suggested "motivated deviance," which I thought would be catchy. (It was several decades before Ziva Kunda [1990] published her paper on "motivated reasoning," so it would not have been title theft.) Ned suggested a more descriptive title, "Opinion divergence as a strategy to avoid being miscast." Not surprisingly, that was the title of the manuscript when it was published (Cooper & Jones, 1969).

Thud. The paper appeared with no notice at all. I am not exaggerating to say that we had hoped that the paper would be picked up by various anthologies of studies. We also imagined it would do what good studies are supposed to do—that is, serve as a target for attack, support, or extension by psychologists who studied attitudes on the one hand, and strategic self-presentation on the other. But it landed with a thud. I can vouch for at least three people having read it (I begged my wife to read it) and occasionally, to this day, I suggest it to my graduate students. I still think the total number of readers hovers around three.

As a purveyor of the journals and a current journal editor, it strikes me that some authors spend as much time thinking of catchy titles as they do about the discussion sections of their manuscripts. The ubiquitous colon separating cute from description (or sometimes cute from cuter) seems to have become an essential aspect of a manuscript. In retrospect, I wish I had spent more time on a title for our opinion divergence article. It might have raised the number of readers at least into double digits.

In the intervening years between then and now, excellent social psychologists have studied attitudes as self-presentation with some intriguingly rich theoretical foundations (e.g., Wilson & Hodges, 1992). Nonetheless, I have often wondered why we were so mistaken about the impact this study would have on the field. I offer two possibilities. One is that we fooled ourselves because of how hard we worked on pulling off the elaborate deception. Perhaps we had placed ourselves in the equivalent of the high-effort condition of Aronson and Mills' (1959) classic effort justification study. We worked so hard that we ended up liking what we did. The second explanation is that titles matter. What you call your research tells interested but overburdened readers whether they should read your article or move on. The moment is soon lost. If readers' eyes do not stop at our entry in the table of contents, they may never look back. Of course, there is a third: that the idea was not as good as we thought, and that remains the possibility that gnaws after all of these years.

The saga of our missed opportunity to make our contribution a highly cited article has a more overarching moral that I offer as advice to new investigators: Follow your interests and do what you love. You, too, may miss an opportunity to splash a cherished idea onto the most-cited list. Perhaps, like mine, it will be because of a wordy title or due to any of a plethora of reasons represented in this volume. On the other hand, there will be another study in your repertoire whose impact you thoroughly underestimated and will become the ubiquitous finding associated with your name. My missed opportunity tells me that, in the end, following your interests wherever they lead will produce more well-known contributions than disappointments. What's in a title? In the short term it may make a difference, but in the long term it is overwhelmed by the substance of your work.

REFERENCES

Aronson, J., & Mills, J. (1959). The effect of severity of initiation on liking for a group. *Journal of Abnormal and Social Psychology, 59*, 177–181.

Cooper, J., & Jones, E. E. (1969). Opinion divergence as a strategy to avoid being miscast. *Journal of Personality and Social Psychology, 13*, 23–30.

Kunda, Z. (1990). The case for motivated reasoning. *Psychological Bulletin, 108*, 480–498.

Wilson, T. D., & Hodges, S. D. (1992). Attitudes as temporary constructions. In L. L. Martin & A. Tesser (Eds.), *The construction of social judgments* (pp. 37–65). Hillsdale, NJ: Erlbaum.

TOM GILOVICH, Cornell University

The Bearable Lightness of Impact

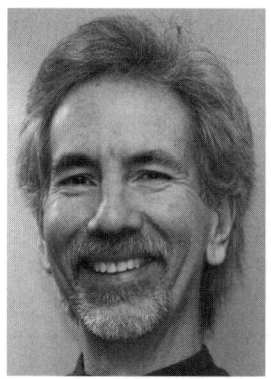

The first paper I ever published examined whether irrelevant features of a decision context can trigger associations to a previous episode and bias how the current decision is approached (Gilovich, 1981). Like many first-time authors, I was naïvely optimistic that the work might receive some attention. For one thing, the paper benefited from unusually wise and helpful feedback from the action editor, Mick Rothhart, who gently led me to cut back the first-timer's tendency to overreach theoretically. The paper also came out at an opportune time: Social psychologists were excited about figuring out how various knowledge structures—schemata, scripts, prototypes, frames, or what Bob Abelson referred to collectively as "things that go bump in the mind"—can be brought to bear on the information people encounter and influence their judgments and decisions. Schank and Abelson's *Scripts, Plans, Goals, and Understanding* (1977) and influential articles by Fiske and Linville (1980) and Taylor and Crocker (1980) gave the subject the aura of an idea whose time was ripe.

There was some existing work demonstrating that constructs planted in the head before information was encountered influenced how that information is processed. The most notable of these, perhaps, was the first of the many "Donald" studies

(Higgins, Rholes, & Jones, 1977). But no paper had yet shown what I set out to explore in the research reported in my first published article. I was interested in how schematic processing of information can sometimes lead to the misapplication of a given schema to a particular decision problem. In one experiment reported in my 1981 paper, National Football League prospects were rated as more likely to excel simply because they came from the same hometown as an established star. In another experiment, a foreign policy crisis was thought to warrant a firmer response if it shared irrelevant similarities to World War II (minorities transported in railroad cars) than if it shared irrelevant similarities to Vietnam (minorities transported in small boats along the coast).

Due to the miracle of self-citation, the paper has actually been referenced in the social psychological literature. But beyond my own efforts to push the work forward, and those of a few kind colleagues, the paper has been ignored. In fact, the most notable attention the paper received was negative. I vividly remember a prominent senior social psychologist during a colloquium visit to Cornell pressing me about what he referred to as "schemagate." What he was concerned about was that, despite all the excited talk about the impact of schemata and how they might bias social information processing, there was no truly solid evidence that this actually ever happened. He told me about lab after lab that had tried and failed to obtain evidence of the sort I had reported and wanted to know, in a tone suggesting a degree of malfeasance worthy of Tricky Dick himself, how I had succeeded when others had not. An unsettling moment for an untenured assistant professor.

With time, of course, we have learned that the senior social psychologist in question needn't have worried about misleading data or false claims. The enormous modern literature on priming contains countless demonstrations of how an activated schema can influence judgments and decisions. Although my own paper on the topic is obscure, its broader point has lived on in spades. In the final analysis, then, it does not matter that that particular paper was consigned to obscurity.

But there may be something interesting to consider by asking why a paper like my initial contribution to the liberature has been ignored when the idea it tried to advance is now such a prominent element of the canon of social psychology. As it turns out, there is a feature of the research I reported that differs from so many of the demonstrations in the priming literature, a feature that might have played a role in the paper's obscurity and, more important, that might speak to something more general about what makes some findings live on and others die out in the marketplace of ideas.

The research I reported could not, by its very nature, match a certain type of clarity and precision that are such enviable features of the typical priming study. If the question is whether an activated construct can distort subsequent information processing more than is normatively defensible, activating the construct via an unrelated prior experience has some obvious advantages. Unscrambling anagrams, finding words in a word search task, or being subliminally exposed to words related to a given construct should not, by any normative accounting, influence the evaluation of stimuli one encounters next. In the typical priming experiment, the event that activates the construct and the to-be-evaluated stimulus are entirely separate and so the former should have absolutely no influence on the latter.

There are occasions, to be sure, in which the sequence played out in the typical priming study does, in fact, occur in everyday life. An encounter with a hostile colleague in the parking lot of the supermarket influences how friendly the clerk at the checkout line seems. Filing a tax return can make another person's charitable contribution seem less altruistic. But these instances notwithstanding, we shouldn't lose sight of the fact that the most common and most powerful engine of schematic processing is not recent activation; it is the fit between elements of a given schema and the features of the stimulus in question. A funeral schema is activated when one sees people wearing black, looking somber, and silently paying attention to a religious official. A hostility schema is activated when one sees that the muscles around everyone's eyes are tight, all smiles have disappeared, and everyone seems on edge, ready for action.

The purpose of my paper was to show that features of a given stimulus that are completely irrelevant to the decision at hand can nonetheless influence a person's response. But it can be a tall order to establish, beyond all doubt, that the shared features truly are irrelevant. It's much easier to make the case that recent activation should have no bearing on the stimulus encountered next. Think of it this way: How many words would be required to summarize an experiment showing that irrelevant features shared by a stored schema and a given stimulus influence how the stimulus is evaluated—and to make it clear that the shared features truly are irrelevant to the task at hand? A lot. Much effort would have to be devoted to an explanation of why the shared features in question should really have no bearing at all on the judgment or decision to be made. Why take the time to do so? Why not simply describe a priming or accessibility study for which the claim that prior exposure in one context should have no bearing on information processing in another context is so much easier to make?

There is an interesting parallel here to the work on the influence of emotional appraisals on judgment. For methodological precision and clarity, it is important to show that an appraisal that accompanies an emotion elicited in one context has a completely unwarranted effect on judgments and decisions in an unrelated context (Lerner & Keltner, 2001). But note that, methodological considerations aside, the most common, pervasive, and important influences of appraisals on judgment are to be found in the very contexts that elicited the emotion in the first place. The sense of certainty that comes with anger distorts one's thinking about the very person who made one mad.

The broader point here is that methodological precision and clarity are, as they should be, important determinants of whether a paper lives on and is often cited. So too is how easily a methodological approach can be summarized and justified. But it is important to keep in mind that the paradigm is not the message; it is only the messenger. And so we should never lose sight of the fact that the phenomena we can study so cleanly with our paradigms are often only a subset of the phenomena, or close cousins of the phenomena, we set out to explore in the first place.

REFERENCES

Fiske, S. T., & Linville, P. W. (1980). What does the schema concept buy us? *Personality and Social Psychology Bulletin, 6,* 543–557.

Gilovich, T. (1981). Seeing the past in the present: The effect of associations to familiar events on judgments and decisions. *Journal of Personality and Social Psychology, 40,* 797–808.

Higgins, E. T., Rholes, W. S., & Jones, C. R. (1977)..Category accessibility and impression formation. *Journal of Experimental Social Psychology, 13,* 141–154.

Lerner, J. S., & Keltner, D. (2001). Fear, anger, and risk. *Journal of Personality and Social Psychology, 81,* 146–159.

Schank, R., & Aberlson, R. P. (1977). *Scripts, plans, goals, and understanding: An inquiry into human knowledge structures.* Hillsdale, NJ: Erlbaum.

Taylor, S. E., & Crocker, J. C. (1980). Schematic bases of social information processing. In E. T. Higgins, P. Herman, & M. P. Zanna (Eds.), *Social cognition: The Ontario symposium* (Vol. 1, pp. 89–134). Hillsdale, NJ: Erlbaum.

JUDITH HARACKIEWICZ, University of Wisconsin

I Can't Explain

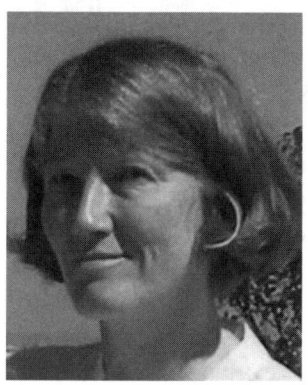

People of a certain generation (yes, I'm "talkin' 'bout my generation") are humming an early song by The Who right now, either "My Generation" or "I Can't Explain." But it was another memorable The Who song that we quoted in one of my earliest papers. I can still remember how excited my graduate students were when they came to show me the results of our first pinball experiment, and how much fun it was to title a paper—"Rewarding pinball wizardry"—and open with lyrics from "Pinball Wizard" from the rock opera *Tommy*. I can still remember my own excitement about working with such great students; for this study, it was George Manderlink and Carol Sansone. We had found an old mechanical pinball machine in the basement of Schermerhorn Hall at Columbia University, rewired it so that we could control participants' scores in a naturalistic manner, and confirmed our suspicion that college students would love playing this antiquated machine. Controversies had been raging about the effects of rewards on intrinsic motivation, and pinball playing seemed the perfect intrinsically motivated behavior to study. Although the early research concerned rewards for task engagement, we were interested in rewards for competence, and such performance-contingent rewards are a lot more complicated. Whenever you reward someone for doing well relative to others, there is the possibility of achieving excellence, symbolized by that reward, but there is also the possibility of feeling pressured or threatened by the performance evaluation implicit in that reward structure.

We argued that rewards for competence might have negative effects due to the stress of performance evaluation, but that they might also have positive effects because they provide positive feedback upon receipt; even more important, they inspire engagement and involvement from the outset as people strive for rewards that symbolize the competence they attain. We tested these ideas with a simple design. In the reward condition, we offered students movie passes for a local theater if their pinball scores were above the 80th percentile, and we ensured that all participants scored well, thereby earning the movie pass. We ran two comparison conditions: (1) in the evaluation condition, we exposed students to performance evaluation relative to the 80th percentile, and told everyone that they scored in the top 20%, and (2) in the feedback-only group, we gave students the same feedback at the conclusion of playing. We measured intrinsic motivation in terms of the number of balls played during a free-time period (and really, how often do you get to have a dependent variable called "balls"?). The results were clear. The evaluation group showed less intrinsic motivation than the feedback-only group, indicating the negative effects of evaluation. The reward group showed more intrinsic motivation than the evaluation group, indicating a positive effect of reward (controlling for the same performance evaluation and feedback), but the same level of intrinsic motivation as the feedback-only group (suggesting that the negative effects of evaluation and positive effects of reward cancelled out). We thought that we had isolated different reward properties with this design, and could explain *why* performance-contingent reward can have both positive and negative effects. We were even naïve enough to think these results might help resolve the raging debate about the effects of rewards on intrinsic motivation.

In hindsight, the results were more complicated than we realized. We could show that performance evaluation was detrimental to intrinsic motivation, and that positive feedback promoted intrinsic motivation, but what conclusion could we draw about the reward effects? These performance-contingent rewards didn't seem to have much effect when compared to feedback-only conditions, but they did promote intrinsic motivation relative to comparable evaluation and feedback, suggesting that there was something special about earning a reward for showing competence. But were these rewards good or bad? There was no easy answer, no bullet summary. Forced to answer a simple question about reward effects, we had to answer with the social psychologist's familiar refrain: "It depends." Social psychologists are rarely interested in main effects or simple conclusions, but rather prefer interactions and conditional conclusions. Indeed, our conclusions depended on the group used for comparison, which made it impossible to categorize this study for the dueling meta-analyses being conducted at the time. Several years later, Carol Sansone and I commented on one controversial meta-analysis by Eisenberger and Cameron (1996) titled, "Detrimental effects of reward: Reality or myth?" with a response titled "Reality is complicated" (Sansone & Harackiewicz, 1998) to highlight the complexity of reward effects.

To muck things up still further, we introduced the term "symbolic cue value" to account for the power of a reward to inspire positive striving toward competence, but failed to convey the importance of this idea, which went against prevailing notions about the detrimental effects of rewards. I really can't explain why we couldn't present this analysis in a more compelling fashion, but I accept full responsibility for using obscure new terms for simple ideas. I think our lack of clarity was compounded by concerns about going against the tide of current thinking. Paralyzed by a desire not to offend the theorists who had inspired us, or held back by political correctness, we seemed unwilling or reluctant to simply state that rewards can be good when they inspire people to strive for excellence. Now, really—how hard was that to explain? And why didn't we say that in 1984? In 2000, Suzanne Hidi and I reviewed the rewards literature and commented on these prevailing opinions: "Furthermore, we consider students who want to excel by trying to be among the best to have maladaptive or politically incorrect goals. Is this not an absurdity?" (Hidi & Harackiewicz, 2000).

Despite our belief that we had identified some critical reward properties, the pinball paper never attracted much attention. I still think it's probably the best experiment I've ever done, even if I can't explain the results clearly 25 years later. I didn't let go of the ideas, and though I haven't used the term "symbolic cue value" much in recent years, I remain interested in how strivings for excellence, even when excellence means outperforming others, can have positive effects on interest and performance. I'm not sure why that should be such a controversial idea. One more thing I can't explain.

REFERENCES

Eisenberger, R., & Cameron, J. (1996). Detrimental effects of reward: Reality or myth? *American Psychologist, 51*, 1153–1166.

Harackiewicz, J. M., Manderlink, G., & Sansone, C. (1984). Rewarding pinball wizardry: Effects of evaluation and cue value on intrinsic interest. *Journal of Personality and Social Psychology, 47*, 287–300.

Hidi, S., & Harackiewicz, J.M. (2000). Motivating the academically unmotivated: A critical issue for the 21st century. *Review of Educational Research, 70*, 151–179.

Sansone, C., & Harackiewicz, J.M. (1998). "Reality" is complicated. Comment on Eisenberger & Cameron. *American Psychologist, 53*, 673–674.

MARK SNYDER, University of Minnesota

Most Underappreciated . . . By Me!

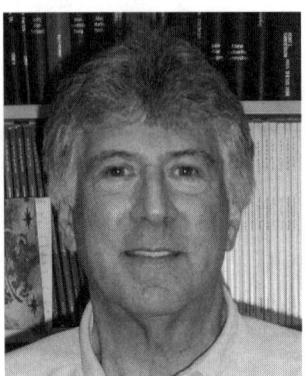

They just don't get it! Who among us has not had that reaction when others seem not to fully appreciate our work? I know that I have felt that way when the reviews of my latest work have been less than ecstatic. And I expect that it's an almost universal reaction, and a quite understandable one. After all, we are in a better position to appreciate our work than anyone else, having been with it every step of the way, having thought long and hard about why the problems that we study are important, why our explanations of our findings work better than alternate explanations, and why our work delivers intellectual benefits to science and practical dividends to society. All of these considerations can and do, and quite naturally, lead to feelings that one's own work is underappreciated by others, who most likely feel that their own work (to which they have given great thought) is underappreciated by us.

Thus, our privileged position vis-à-vis our own work may set the stage for us to feel that our work is underappreciated by others. But I believe that there is another form of underappreciation of our own work: by ourselves. But this underappreciation of our own work may not be immediately apparent; it may only emerge over time as we realize that there may be "more than meets the eye" in our own work.

Let me speak from the perspective of one of my own experiences of underappreciating my work, and how I grew to appreciate it more fully over time.

For many years, my colleagues and I have investigated the ways in which expectations influence the course of social interaction. Typically, in these studies, two people who have never met before have a brief getting-acquainted conversation, with one member of the pair (referred to as the "perceiver") being given an expectation about the other person (known as the "target"). Typically, in these interactions, perceivers act as if their expectations were true, and targets come to behave as if the expectations were in fact true. For example, in an early study of behavioral confirmation in social interaction, when perceivers had a telephone conversation with targets they believed to be physically attractive (as a result of seeing a photo ostensibly of the target, but actually chosen by random assignment), those targets came to behave in more friendly, outgoing, and sociable ways than targets interacting with perceivers who believed them to be physically unattractive, with these differences in the behavior of the target being readily apparent to outside observers who listen in on the target's contributions to the conversations and know nothing at all about the perceiver's expectations (Snyder, Tanke, & Berscheid, 1977).

This "behavioral confirmation" scenario (so named because the behavior of the target comes to confirm the expectations of the perceiver in the course of their social interaction) has been demonstrated for a wide range of expectations (including beliefs about personality, ability, gender, race) and a variety of interaction contexts (including relatively unstructured interactions such as initial getting-acquainted conversations between strangers as well as relatively structured interactions such as those between teachers and students and between counselors and clients); for a review, see Snyder (1992). On first consideration, the formula for behavioral confirmation seems to be a quite straightforward one: perceiver + expectation + target = behavioral confirmation. Given that behavioral confirmation could be readily observed in a social interaction as seemingly simple as a brief, unstructured telephone conversation, with perceivers and targets not being required to do anything other than get acquainted with each other, it did seem that behavioral confirmation was the "natural" and "automatic" consequence of people interacting in the context of expectations, something that might routinely (even if not inevitably) occur whenever people meet others about whom they have expectations.

Yet, as much as the facts of the behavioral confirmation scenario are simple and straightforward, and as much as it seems that behavioral confirmation just "happens" when perceivers and targets are put together, it has turned out that it's not quite that simple, and there appears to be a much more complicated dynamic in play in the interactions that culminate in behavioral confirmation. Research on the necessary and sufficient conditions for behavioral confirmation to occur, as well as research on its underlying mechanisms, tells us that the behavioral confirmation scenario requires a fairly elaborate coordination of the agendas of perceiver and target, with both parties to the interaction actively involved in pursuing quite different approaches to pursuing the goal of getting acquainted with each other (for a review, see Snyder [1992]). The *perceiver*, it turns out, views interaction as an opportunity to *get to know* the target, to find out if the expectation fits and whether it serves well to predict what the target will be like and as a useful guide to how to handle the interaction. The way that the perceiver pursues that agenda for action is a "confirmatory" one of giving targets opportunities to behave in accord with expectations more so than opportunities to contradict the expectation. The *target*, on the other hand, views interaction as an opportunity to *get along* with the perceiver, to find a way to ensure a smooth and pleasing flow of interaction, and uses the perceiver's overtures as cues to how to handle the interaction and thus goes along with the perceiver's overtures, which has the effect of confirming the perceiver's expectations.

Adding even more complexity and nuance to the portrait of behavioral confirmation, it appears that these contrasting, but interlocking, agendas can be (and often are) exacerbated by power differences between perceivers and targets. Often, it is persons in positions of power who hold expectations (teachers of their students, employers of their workers, therapists of their clients) and have the power of their roles to pursue an agenda that involves acting on expectations about the target and leading the target to provide behavioral confirmation. By contrast, targets of expectations, especially those related to stereotyped beliefs and prejudicial attitudes, are often members of disadvantaged and powerless stigmatized groups, having little option other than to pursue agendas of going along with the overtures of those in power and confirming their expectations. And research has indicated that a power differential, in which the perceiver holds more power than the target, is necessary for behavioral confirmation to occur (e.g., Copeland, 1994), a power differential that can come from the roles that perceivers and targets often occupy (e.g., Snyder & Klein, 2005) and that can emerge from the very holding of expectations and the advantage of knowing more about the target than the target knows about the perceiver (e.g., Baldwin, Kiviniemi, & Snyder, 2009).

Thus, to think of behavioral confirmation being something that "just happens" when perceivers interact with the targets of their expectations is to underappreciate the complexity of the phenomenon. I will confess that, for quite some time, I thought of behavioral confirmation as something that just happened when social interactions occurred under the cover of expectations, with the reality of expectations somehow "spreading" from the mind of the perceiver to the behavior of the target. To some extent, the appeal of thinking in such terms may reflect one of my original goals for research on behavioral confirmation, namely to show that beliefs make a difference, that they aren't just things that reside in people's mind, confined to the world of thought. Indeed, research on the behavioral confirmation did reveal that beliefs don't operate in a vacuum; to the contrary, in the course of social interaction, they affect how people act, how they treat other people, and how other people in turn behave. My interests in such "social constructivist" themes are longstanding, having been nurtured by my studies as an undergraduate at McGill University, as a doctoral student at Stanford University, and as a member of the faculty at the University of Minnesota. However, given the apparent simplicity of the research paradigm (two people getting acquainted, one of whom holds an expectation about the other), it was quite easy to slip into thinking that behavioral confirmation was something that just happened as expectations spread from the mind of the perceiver to the behavior or the target.

Thinking that way was, of course, to underappreciate all that can and does go on under the surface of two people meeting and getting acquainted, one of whom holds an expectation about what the other person is like. Of course, it has taken a considerable amount of research, involving experimental manipulations to system-atically influence the agendas of perceivers and targets and to systematically create differential balances of power between perceiver and target, to document the successive steps in the chain of events that occur when people bring preconceived beliefs and expectations to their interactions with other people. From that research has come a fuller appreciation (certainly by me, and I hope by others) of the complex intertwining of belief and reality in social interaction.

But I will confess that that there has been a price associated with getting rid of my own underappreciation of all that goes into the behavioral confirmation scenario. Knowing that behavioral confirmation requires the convergence of inter-locking agendas of perceivers and targets in the context of power differentials that facilitate the enactment of those agendas takes some of the "mystique" and the "magic" out of the behavioral confirmation phenomenon. So, am I nostalgic for my earlier underappreciation of the complexity of behavioral confirmation? And do I think that others would prefer that things had stayed simple, and we had not progressed beyond a "put two people together with an expectation and it will happen" view of behavioral confirmation? No, not really, as the "demystification" of the phenomenon that comes with the understanding of the mechanisms does seem to be the price to be paid for a better scientific understanding of the phenomenon, and that would seem to be a price well worth paying. Certainly, it has been for me, and I hope it can and will be for other investigators as well.

REFERENCES

Baldwin, A. S., Kiviniemi, M. T., & Snyder, M. (2009). A subtle source of power: The effect of having an expectation on anticipated interpersonal power. *Journal of Social Psychology, 149*, 82–104.

Copeland, J. T. (1994). Prophecies of power: Motivational implications of social power for behavioral confirmation. *Journal of Personality and Social Psychology, 67*, 264–277.

Snyder, M. (1992). Motivational foundations of behavioral confirmation. *Advances in Experimental Social Psychology, 25*, 67–114.

Snyder, M., & Klein, O. (2005). Construing and constructing others: On the reality and the generality of the behavioral confirmation scenario. *Interaction Studies, 6*, 53–67.

Snyder, M., Tanke, E. D., & Berscheid, E. (1977). Social perception and interpersonal behavior: On the self-fulfilling nature of social stereotypes. *Journal of Personality and Social Psychology, 35*, 656–666.

JOHN F. DOVIDIO, Yale University

It Takes More Than Two to Tango: The Importance of Identifying and Addressing Your Audience

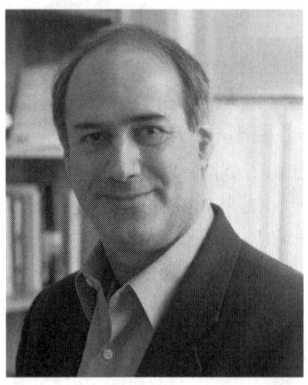

In the early 1980s, I published two empirical papers with Sam Gaertner, my dissertation advisor and now longtime collaborator, that were stimulated by ongoing political debates and growing resistance in public opinion and political action against affirmative action (Dovidio & Gaertner, 1981, 1983). The political landscape of race relations had been volatile over the previous two decades. The 1960s were characterized by landmark changes, politically and legally, in race relations in the United States. The civil rights legislation of the mid-1960s outlawed a broad range of traditional discriminatory policies and practices. Racial discrimination was no longer simply a moral issue, it was a legal one. The legislation in the late 1960s establishing affirmative action went even further. It was designed to reverse the adverse effects of historical discrimination on Blacks and several other traditionally disadvantaged groups, including women. By the late 1970s, however, the social and political pendulum was beginning to swing the other way. In *Regents of California v. Bakke*, the Supreme Court in 1978 limited the scope of affirmative action programs, essentially banning racial quotas.

The debates surrounding the Bakke case helped crystallize our research focus. We noted, "Although recent protests by whites regarding affirmative action seem to articulate only the concern that qualified whites will be subordinated to *less qualified* blacks . . ., it is possible that the reversal traditional role relationship itself represents the primary threat to whites" (Dovidio & Gaertner, 1981, p. 192). We tested this idea with a laboratory analogue. In the first study (Dovidio & Gaertner, 1981), White participants interacted with a Black or White male confederate who was introduced as either their supervisor or subordinate and as either higher or lower (ostensibly based on a pretest) in cognitive ability to themselves. Participants' responses of interest included a spontaneous measure of helping, assisting the confederate pick up pencils that he "accidentally" knocked over, and evaluations of the confederate and the self.

We found, as expected, that status, not ability, affected how positively White participants behaved toward the Black confederate. Regardless of the level of ability, participants responded less positively to the Black confederate when he was their supervisor than their subordinate. Moreover, although participants recognized that the higher-ability Black was more competent than the lower-ability Black, they still rated themselves as at least as competent as the higher-ability Black confederate. Thus, participants accepted that a Black person could be quite competent, but not more competent than themselves. Consequently, they questioned the fairness of having any Black supervisor. When the confederate was White, however, participants acknowledged the greater competence of the higher-ability confederate, and they responded more positively to him, in helping and in evaluations, than to the lower-ability White confederate. In a subsequent study (Dovidio & Gaertner, 1983), we conceptually replicated these results using White female and male confederates instead of Black and White male confederates. Both male and female participants responded less favorably to female than to male supervisors, regardless of their ability. We concluded that people may resist implementations of affirmative action because, perhaps without their full awareness, they are threatened by being subordinated to Blacks and women.

When we published these two papers, four and six years after I earned my PhD, I was very optimistic about the attention the work would receive. The work was timely politically, and within the field of social psychology racial prejudice, sexism, and helping behavior were very active topics of study. The work, I believed, was destined to receive broad attention and stimulate more research on this conceptually and practically important topic. I was wrong. The 1981 article was cited six times over the next decade by other researchers; the 1983 paper was first cited in 1995. Rather than recognition or, perhaps, controversy, the reaction was one of scholarly indifference.

In retrospect, several different factors likely contributed to the underappreciation of this pair of publications. Part of the problem was poor timing. In 1981, when Ronald Reagan assumed the presidency of the United States, the politics of the United States took a conservative shift. During the Reagan administration, affirmative action was systematically restricted legislatively and judicially. In the realm of public opinion, the arguments for resistance to affirmative action focus on perceived flaws in the policy, not on the psychology of the dominant group. The public and the media had little interest in an argument, empirical or not, that racism and sexism might fundamentally underlie resistance to affirmative action and other programs to address and compensate for individual and structural discrimination.

However, given the still-prevalent liberal leanings of academics, the wave of political conservativism nationally is not likely a full explanation of the lack of scholarly impact of the papers. The main problems were rooted in decisions I made as an author and researcher. I was a freshly-minted PhD, and a bit impetuous. Although Sam Gaertner was a co-author on this work, I wanted to take primary responsibility for shepherding this research into the literature. I made two mistakes, though. The first was framing the paper too diffusely. The second was my inappropriate placement of the work.

With 25 more years of experience under my belt, coupled with the general benefits of hindsight, I now recognize that I framed the manuscript too broadly. Currently, when I sit down with collaborators to begin writing a paper, the first question I ask is: What's the story? I now understand that I need to present a clear, focused, and compelling exposition to readers that captures their interest and guides them effortlessly along in a linear, logical path. From the very beginning, the message of the 1981 paper lacked a singular focus. The article was titled, "The effects of race, status and ability on helping behavior," but it began with a broad discussion of the Bakke decision, the consideration of the Kerner Commission Report on civil unrest in the 1960s, and a review of public opinion about social policy. Thus, the title might attract a reader interested in the dynamics of pro-social behavior, but the first page of the article had little to say about the topic. Readers who might be interested in the political debates that stimulated the work would be unlikely, based on the title, to pick out the article to read. Basically, the article was written in a way designed more to please me, the author, than to attract or please other readers. The extended discussion of affirmative action and public opinion chronicled how my ideas for the research developed, but it did little to directly elucidate the psychological dynamics of pro-social motivation. I made the emphasis of the work the evolution of the ideas that stimulated it rather than the final central message of the work itself; this *was* the story, to me, but it detracted from the story I needed to tell the reader. Then, to compound the problem, the 1983 article used a parallel title, "The effects of sex, status and ability on helping behavior," and began once again with a discussion of protests against affirmative action. And when the focus of the introduction finally shifted to helping behavior, the emphasis was on conceptually replicating the results of the 1981 paper. If the original article attracted only a limited audience, it should be no surprise that a conceptual replication of the original finding would attract an even smaller audience.

With respect to the issue of article placement, it is important to note that before electronic abstracting, the journal in which an article was published was even more important for reaching an appropriate audience than it is today. People normally subscribed to a limited number of journals, which they received only in hard copy, and they typically visually scanned the table of contents of these journals to identify relevant works. The 1981 race and helping paper was originally submitted to the top journal in social psychology. The reviews were thorough and helpful. One was very positive—still today the most favorable review I have ever received on a manuscript—but the other one was mixed. The editor invited a revision. However, by the time the paper was revised and resubmitted, a new editor had assumed the leadership of the journal and that editor decided, without outside review or consultation, to reject the manuscript. I was confused and devastated. I decided to send it back out to another highly respected journal, *Social Psychology Quarterly*. This journal had a strong citation impact factor, it was a flagship journal of the American Sociological Association, and one of my earlier papers there had received considerable attention. My submission received positive reviews there, and with minor additional revision it was accepted.

The problem was that although articles in *Social Psychology Quarterly* were generally well cited, few studies of helping behavior were published in the journal. Moreover, most of the prosocial behavior studies that were published in there involved field methods and focused on non-spontaneous forms of helping, such a donating and volunteering, that addressed current sociological theories related to community functioning, social movements, and activism. A laboratory experiment of a spontaneous and basically trivial form was ill suited for the journal's primary audience, sociologists. Also, around this time, the number of psychologically-oriented social psychologists who submitted and subscribed to the journal was beginning to decline as new social psychological journals were beginning to emerge in the discipline. When coupled with the problem of the diffuse framing of the article itself, the paper seemed destined to be lost to the intended audience, experimental social psychologists interested in helping and/or race. The articles that appeared immediately before and after our paper, both much more traditionally sociological in their approach, were cited much more frequently. Furthermore, because I was eager to get another publication on my *vita* before I came up for tenure, the 1983 paper was sent to a respectable but not top-tier journal, with limited circulation. The framing of this paper was not compelling enough to attract scholarly attention beyond what other papers in the journal normally garnered. As a consequence, both papers have languished in the archives of psychological research.

Of course, one interpretation of the history of these two papers is that they are not really *under*appreciated but rather appropriately appreciated (given their quality)! Nevertheless, from the favorable comments I received from reviewers, I believe that these two articles were scientifically rigorous and did have something valuable to contribute. Moreover, they have stood the test of time rather well, compared to their initial impact. These two papers were cited more in the past three years than in the first 10-year periods after they were published. Although the contribution of these studies to the advancement of my career was more modest than I hoped, I learned two valuable professional lessons. First, work needs to be framed clearly and economically in a way that meets readers' needs and interests (not necessarily the author's). Papers need to focus on the immediate message of the data, not on the researcher's conceptual journey that originally stimulated the line of work. Second, outlets need to be assessed in terms of their immediate and potential future readership, not solely on prestige or impact factors. Quality of a journal is, of course, a primary consideration. However, among journals of comparable quality it is important to determine which has the audience that will be most receptive to an article's method and message. And, today, even that may be obscured by the fact that most of what people know about a topic is found in electronic literature searches, anyway, where a search engine such as PsycInfo finds everything. The key to being found, and read, then, may be "keywords" in the characterization of one's work, rather than the location of its publication. In the end, I learned that publication is not primarily about me or my career, but instead it should be about disseminating scientific knowledge, which requires identifying, attracting, and meeting the needs of readers. Thus, the goal should not be simply to publish; rather, it should be to *communicate*—and to identify, and communicate to, the appropriate audience.

REFERENCES

Dovidio, J. F., & Gaertner, S. L. (1981). The effects of race, status and ability on helping behavior. *Social Psychology Quarterly, 44,* 192–203.
Dovidio, J. F., & Gaertner, S. L. (1983). The effects of sex, status, and ability on helping behavior. *Journal of Applied Social Psychology, 13,* 191–205.

DAVID DUNNING, Cornell University

My Rather Unknown Piece About "Unknown Unknowns" and Their Role in Self-Insight

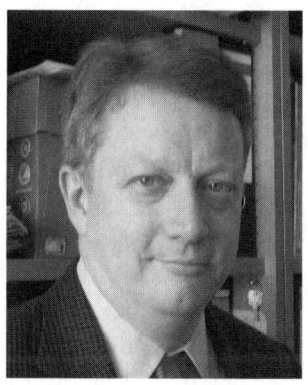

Imagine you lived the life of a person suffering from hemiagnosia. People with this condition, caused by damage to one hemisphere of the brain, possess no awareness of half their visual world. Their eyes report the proper visual data to the brain, but they are unable to throw their spotlight of attention to one side, usually the left side, of the environment. As such, they may shave only one side of their face or eat only half the food on their plate, even if they complain of hunger. But here's the trick. In the mind of hemiagnosic people, their world is just as full as ours is to us. They are not aware of missing anything, save for an occasional bump into furniture.

But here's the other trick. In a metaphorical sense, when it comes to problem solving, all of us already metaphorically live in the world of the hemiagnosic, in that there is potentially a lot of knowledge and expertise that lies outside our ken. The doctor might not know all the treatments that should be considered; the detective might miss important clues at a crime scene. Thus, although people may have exquisitely accurate understanding of the knowledge they use to tackle some program, much like hemiagnosic patients, they likely have no awareness of just how much further knowledge they remain ignorant of.

In a sense, this observation that there is information and expertise beyond our awareness is not new. In 2002, Secretary of Defense William Rumsfeld, in his description of the challenges facing antiterrorism efforts, infamously noted that there were many known terrorism risks in the world (i.e., "known knowns," as he termed them), but that there were also known risks that he had incomplete information on—something he termed "known unknowns." However, he observed that the most worrying problem for national security was a different type of risk—risks that were real but that fell outside the imagination of the national security community. "Unknown unknowns" was how he labeled them.

The reaction of the press was to guffaw at Secretary Rumsfeld and his presumably sophist allocution about unknown unknowns, but any engineer will tell you this is an important idea that keeps him or her up at night. Engineers and designers know that their structures and devices often contain "unk unks," as they are affectionately known, and it is these unk unks that more often than not cause their creations to fail. This concern, for example, causes architects, after taking special care to calculate just how much concrete they need to ensure that a building will be stable, to use eight times that amount in the actual building.

In 2005, Deanna Caputo and I published a paper designed to explore the role of unknown unknowns in the realm of self-evaluation. We knew from past research that people really do not do a good job at evaluating their knowledge and expertise. Often, people hold flattering opinions of their competence that are not backed by objective evidence or that are statistically plausible (for a review, see Dunning [2005]). We wondered if people achieved such lackluster accuracy because they were not aware of unk unks—in this case, possible solutions to problems that lay outside their knowledge. Our paper contained five experiments designed to see if people showed any awareness of relevant unknown unknowns or gave them any weight in self-evaluations. For example, one experiment asked participants to provide as many solutions to a word puzzle as they could. In another, graduate students were presented with flawed research studies and asked to enumerate all the methodological and statistical flaws they found.

Across the studies, a clear picture emerged: Participants showed little insight into the scope of their ignorance—and this ignorance of ignorance was a major contributor to mistaken self-evaluations. When judging their performance, participants gave great weight to the number of solutions they had found in the problems we gave them, but none to the number they had missed—even though they conceded that this last statistic was relevant. Indeed, their estimates about how many solutions they had missed usually bore no relationship to the truth. But, once made aware of those solutions, and thus the scope of their ignorance, participants gave substantial weight to these misses and, more important, they became more accurate and less flattering in their self-judgments. In short, people were eager to incorporate missed solutions into their self-evaluations. However, unless those solutions were explicitly pointed out to them, participants showed no ability to intuit the range and number of these unknown unknown solutions.

I would love to report what the reaction of the research community has been to this article—except there really has not been any. As I am writing this, only two other scholars have cited this work, suggesting that the research community would find it perfectly acceptable if this paper had stayed in the realm of the unknown unpublished. This non-reaction is notable for two reasons. First, when I describe this study to non-academics, they tend to find it thought-provoking and valuable. The paper is something of a "hit" to a lay audience.

Second, Dunning and Caputo (2005) is merely a generalization of a point made in the most cited and celebrated article I have ever been involved with. In Kruger and Dunning (1999), we pointed out that incompetent people—those *really* lacking knowledge and expertise—suffer a double curse. First, their shortcomings cause them to make many mistakes. Second, these exact same shortcomings rob them of the ability to realize they are making mistakes and that other people are choosing more wisely. Kruger and Dunning (1999), although it describes only a special case within the Caputo and Dunning framework, has enjoyed a different professional fate: It has been cited over 300 times, has been featured in several popular newspapers and magazines, has provided the context for a *Doonesbury* cartoon, has inspired theater pieces, and has been even christened the "Dunning–Kruger effect" in the blogosphere.[1]

Thus, a central question for me is why Kruger and Dunning (1999) is so notorious when Caputo and Dunning (2005) is so ignored—given that they make roughly equivalent points about human ignorance. In all, I can think of three reasons for the latter paper's fate. First, to my regret, the main point of Caputo and Dunning can be twisted just a bit to sound banal; all that it shows is that people do not know what they do not know. In the review process for publication, several reviewers had this reaction, and as a consequence yawned as they rejected it.

What the reviewers did not get, and what we really tried to emphasize, was that the headline was really something else. Even if we concede that our basic insight was banal, at least one very important implication is not. If people do not—strike that, cannot—anticipate the scope of their ignorance, we can draw one simple conclusion about accurate self-evaluation: It is nearly *impossible*. If accurately knowing one's self means knowing how much one does not know, then people are just not in possession of crucial information they need to evaluate themselves accurately. Their *information environment* (Dunning, 2005) is inadequate. That said, the same complaint about banality can be leveled at Kruger and Dunning (1999). So why did Kruger and Dunning avoid this critique? I think it did because the phenomenon it described is so very visible in everyday life. An incompetent person clueless about his or her competence is a person we have all rolled our eyes at. The Dunning–Kruger effect makes itself quite known in our everyday lives flamboyantly.

The phenomenon described in Caputo and Dunning (2005) may be more pervasive, but it slinks around more invisibly. We often do not see when we—or others—have hit the limits of personal knowledge. In at least one circumstance in my life, the phenomenon is interesting because it exactly leads people to render it invisible. One of the ironies of being a college professor is that student advisees who most need my advice never show up to obtain it. These are the students who do not realize that there are questions they need to ask, preparations they must make, tasks they have to do, and advice they had better seek out. Because they never bother to show up at my office, their ignorance remains invisible—to them and to me. Paradoxically, the students who do show up to my office are those bright enough to know that there must be something they do not know. Of course, they are also the ones smart enough to know how to go about finding out on their own what that something is. These students are exactly those most primed to take up my advice; they just do not need it, showing up at my office just to check their work. However, let me add, gentle reader, that if you are a student, you may not necessarily know which of the above groups you fall into, and so it might be best just to check in once in a while.

The final, most significant, reason I believe the Caputo and Dunning (2005) phenomenon is neglected is because its main point fails as a piece of gossip. Just like everyone else in everyday life, psychologists are just people who trade gossip about what remarkable things people do in our labs. Our stories might contain more quantification and precision, but in the end we are storytellers regaling each other with tales of people's conduct while under our observation.

The key is that gossip is most fun when it puts the focus on *people*. The Dunning–Kruger effect has bushels of gossip value because focuses on certain types of people (i.e., the incompetent) and the remarkable things they do (i.e., "You won't believe those clueless people had no idea about how bad they were doing!"). Caputo and Dunning (2005), however, focuses not on people but rather the task they face. Our major take-away message was that the *task* of self-evaluation is impossible. But in focusing on the task, we robbed our findings of its gossip value. It is hard to gossip about a task, (e.g., "Hey, do you want to know what self-evaluation did last week?").

This leads me to wonder that, perhaps, as researchers, our stories focus too much on people and fail to gossip enough about the task demands they face. Think about how many "heuristics," "effects," and "phenomena" in the literature are defined in terms of people's actions rather than on situational parameters that may pull for those actions. To be sure, it is only human, in explaining social behavior, to place the emphasis on people and their quirks and frailties, while at the same time giving short shrift to the situations or task demands. There are even a couple of names for this in the literature: *correspondence bias* and the *fundamental attribution error*. But I think we are too quick to blame (or praise) people for their actions in our experiments, and too slow to recognize how task demands might really be the causal agents that produce the behavior we see.

Consider, for example, the task of self-evaluation. One should not quickly blame people for erroneous self-impressions. People might strive to reach accurate self-insight, but the world makes it difficult to achieve it. Feedback is sparse, imperfect, ambiguous, and often hidden. Other people seem averse to telling us what they really think about us, often flattering to deceive. And then there are all those unk unks. In such an environment, it is not a surprise that people are so often wrong about themselves (Dunning, 2005).

Thus, if there is an "unknown unknown" opportunity that I think we researchers miss, it is the chance to recast our findings not in terms of human tendencies but more in terms of what task or situational demands make possible or impossible. Do not focus on why people stereotype; instead, consider why the task of avoiding stereotypes is so difficult. Do not blame people for their imperfect memories; ask instead why accurate memories are hard to keep. For myself, this has become a basic question I always ask: What is it in the environment that I can blame for this apparently human shortcoming? By thinking this way, we might shrink, at least a little, the scope of our own metaphorical hemiagnosia.

NOTE

1. It remains a mystery why the blogosphere switched the order of our names in labeling the effect. I hope it is not a comment on the comparative incompetence Justin and I have somewhere exhibited.

REFERENCES

Caputo, D. D., & Dunning, D. (2005). What you don't know: The role played by errors of omission in imperfect self-assessments. *Journal of Experimental Social Psychology, 41,* 488–505.

Dunning, D. (2005). *Self-insight: Roadblocks and detours on the path to knowing thyself.* New York: Psychology Press.

Kruger, J. M., & Dunning, D. (1999). Unskilled and unaware of it: How difficulties in recognizing one's own incompetence lead to inflated self-assessments. *Journal of Personality and Social Psychology, 77,* 1121–1134.

MICHAEL HARRIS BOND, Polytechnic University of
Hong Kong

Reality Lives! Redeeming an Apparently Unfulfilled Prophecy

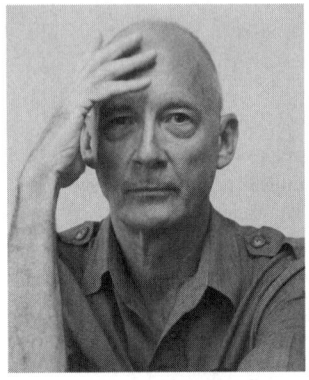

> I don't like work . . . but I like what is in work—the chance to find yourself, your own
> reality—for yourself, not for others—which no other man can ever know.
>
> Joseph Conrad, *The Heart of Darkness*

As he watched me waltz out the door in the heat of a summer Saturday night, my dad used to sigh, "Oh son, if only I could be your age and know what I know now." I might well say the same about my PhD and its subsequent incarnations, both in print (Bond, 1972, 1987) and, more importantly for this professionally uncertain soul, in the heart-mind of my colleagues.

Over the ensuing 40 years, I have retained a keen affection for this early work, perhaps because I have never been closer to the matrix of the data it yielded. I planned the study myself, having recently lost my PhD advisor to a mid-career crisis the year before graduation, recruited and ran my subjects (as they were then known), hand-scored the person-perception data from questionnaires and extracted nonverbal indicators from the video records of the interaction between my participant pairs, analyzed the results on a handheld Casio calculator, wrote up the study during my postdoctoral year, and finalized my submission to *JPSP* from distant Japan, where competent typists for my academic English were difficult to find—without a spell-check provided by Word (this was 1971), I found my proofreading skills stretched to the max! Seymour Rosenberg then shepherded my submission to eventual publication with consideration and a level of professionalism that has set a personal standard for me to emulate in my subsequent editing work. So, I might well have been satisfied with its eventual publication in our premier outlet, right?

No. Over the years, I was disappointed that its surprising results were not cited more frequently, a surprise probably shared by most of us to the reception accorded our first-born solo efforts. But there was more to my discontent: Something irritated me about the way I had represented the participants' actions and experience through my glib use of terms like "self-reversing prophecy." This term made sense from the perspective of the scientist eager to join a chorus of researchers on a fascinating topic, but it did not feel true to how my participants (Stanford students like me, after all!) grappled with the experimental challenge that I had presented them. It took me 15 years to satisfy my sense of integrity as a behavioral scientist and gain a sense of closure on my thesis research. So what was I obsessing about over those long years?

THE MISE-EN-SCENE

In 1967, I took Walter Mischel's mind-jolting course in personality, where he required us to read galley proofs of his forthcoming *Personality and Assessment* (1968). Personality, as a defensible topic of study, appeared to disappear before my mind's eye, since its trans-situational consistency could not be empirically demonstrated. But why then, I wondered, did us normal folks continue to believe in the apparent fiction that we and other persons were the same persons across the situations of our lives? I had a flash, endorsed by Dr. Mischel (we addressed our teachers using honorifics in the 1960s!) in his reactions to my class paper: Perhaps we social actors develop an impression of another person for whatever reasons, then act towards that person in a way that makes his or behavior conform to our impression, rendering others consistent to our mind's eye. I proposed that we may create and sustain the interpersonal reality that surrounds us.

Understandably, then, encountering Rosenthal and Jacobson's aptly named *Pygmalion in the Classroom* (1968) left me inspired. This study reported that, on average, the IQs of primary students in San Mateo County increased over the course of a school year if they were described as "bloomers" to their teachers at the beginning of that school year. True, the effect was not big, and it declined in size from the first to the sixth grade, but nonetheless I was amazed that a person could be so "shapeable" by another person's holding a mere impression of him or her, and on such an important psychological attribute as intelligence. Were we all Henry Higginses, shaping the Eliza Doolittles in our interpersonal networks?

The media lionized the findings as evidence for dangerous, stereotype-confirming prophecies in the nation's very educational cradle, lending the findings an even greater weight in my impressionable mind. Mark Snyder, a year behind me in the Stanford PhD program, soon thereafter put together a series of remarkable studies confirming the operation of self-fulfilling prophecies in other domains of social interaction (these studies are subsequently summarized in Snyder & Stukas [1999]). Such engaging reading, especially for those of us raised in a Promethean cultural orientation! They became "must-includes" in our social psychology texts, and still are. The self-fulfilling prophecy had entered our discipline as a taken-for-granted staple on our intellectual menu.

A SELF-REVERSING PROPHECY

Unfortunately, perhaps, I (Bond, 1972) found quite the opposite of a self-fulfilling prophecy. Students, primed to think that their future conversational partner was "cold," behaved more warmly as rated by independent judges when chatting with that partner than when that same partner had been described to another conversational partner as "warm." The "cold-primed" conversational partners reciprocated by acting more warmly than their "warm-primed" comparison partners; they even smiled more! This result constituted a reversal, not a fulfillment, of interpersonal prophecy.

It was, of course, unexpected, and I don't think that I provided a compelling explanation for the outcome, *ex post facto*. Nor did I, a timid neophyte, give the paper a "zinger" title, like "Reversing the self-fulfilling prophecy–disconfirmation lives!," that might have piqued scholarly interest. Further, those social psychologists who might have read the abstract found themselves confronting a counterintuitive finding without a theoretical lifeline to guide them through the maze. And of course, I suspect that most of us want to believe in self-fulfilling prophecies, as it accords with the Horatio Alger dynamic that makes sense of our own personal successes in individualistic cultural traditions—we *can* make the world dance to our projections! So, my first solo paper fell beneath the intellectual horizon, having failed to confirm our disciplinary expectations. According to Google Scholar, it has been cited only 22 times since its publication 37 years ago.

Even with the subsequent discoveries of "behavioral disconfirmation" by Bill Ickes and Mark Snyder, combined with heroic attempts to embed both confirmation and disconfirmation effects within a broader framework (Snyder & Stukas, 1999), the pull of self-fulfilling prophecies continues. Searching Google Scholar recently for "behavioral confirmation," I found 241,000 hits, compared to 21,500 for "behavioral disconfirmation"—an 11:1 ratio. Perhaps Francis Bacon was right in averring, "When any proposition has been once laid down, the human understanding forces everything else to add fresh support and confirmation . . . rather than sacrifice the authority of its first conclusions" (Bacon, 1620/2000, Aphorism 46). Our discipline's first conclusion had been that behavioral confirmation was the typical outcome from social interactions, and the rest was fine-tuning.

THE SENTIENT PARTICIPANT

What I found irritating about this intellectual interplay among us social psychologists was the neglect of our participants' experience following the "prophetic" exchange of which he or she was the primary architect. Rather, the focus had been upon the target of the prophecy, the labeled other. I had earlier tried to generate prophetic impact in two carefully designed and executed experiments, but to no discernible effect. Could social reality be less malleable than our skillfully orchestrated demonstrations (that made their way into print!) were suggesting? Was there a "reality" to the other person about whom we may hold an impression that no amount of scientific necromancy could shift, the ballast of, egads, the other's "personality" that could not be easily shifted? Was there perhaps a reality to the other that we were overlooking in our social psychological "rush to judgment" that endorsed the ubiquity of self-fulfilling prophecies?

Testing such possibilities requires that the experimenter allow the participants holding the impression to "speak," assessing changes in their impression of the subsequent interaction partner before *and* after their interaction, then correlating the degree of impression change with some objective measure of partner personality revealed during that interaction. I had these measures but had not fully used them in the original publication; I had been focusing on my experimenter's perspective, using the pre-interaction measure of the future interaction partner merely as a manipulation check. I had thereafter ignored the participant's perspective on the ensuing event; all was focused on whether the prophecy about the prophet's partner had been fulfilled or not.

Refocusing on the impression holder, however, I found considerable change in each prophesier's ratings of her partner's warmth, especially in the experimental condition where she believed her future partner to be cold. Her judged warmth of the "cold" target increased dramatically; that of the "warm" target decreased slightly. In both cases, the degree of change closely tracked the revealed level of warmth displayed by the partner, as rated by independent judges of the interaction. Apparently (and can one believe appearances?), the initial impression of warmth or coldness shaped by my experimental manipulation had anchored the impression holder's belief about the partner. However, this belief had shifted in close correspondence to the partner's independently judged warmth as revealed during the subsequent interaction. Prophets were thus responding sensitively to the revealed warmth of their labeled partner. Reality lives!

A MATTER OF PERSPECTIVE

The interaction had not completely eliminated the original difference in warmth that I had successfully manipulated in the fresh minds of my impression holders. From their perspective, the experimenter-induced impression had been fulfilled—"warm" partners were still warmer than "cold" partners at the end of these encounters; from the experimenter's perspective and using the ratings from the independent judges, the initial impressions had been reversed. Of course, I had only tracked one interaction, and that was from the outset of the relationship between my two participants. What would happen over the course of future exchanges? Would the prophet's impression eventually be whittled down and come to match that of the objective judges, providing full support to the notion of a shared social reality concerning the personality of the other person? Or would some intransigent shard of the original manipulated impression remain, confirming Bacon's 17th-century claim?

Such work remains to be done, though I expect that it never will; it's not jazzy enough and would require a time- and resource-consuming longitudinal design to address. For my part, I was content to have shown to my own satisfaction that our experimental participants, folks like us after all, paid close attention to the social reality with which they were engaged; they, and we, tested reality and assessed the feedback we received. This feedback, like journal and chapter reviews, channeled our responses to our initial gambits, and we altered our original impressions and ripostes accordingly, though perhaps not completely (there's probably some facet of personality that shapes if and how we respond to interpersonal feedback—"other monitoring," perhaps?).

Having reanalyzed my original data from Bond (1972), I wrote up the article described above and submitted it to *Social Cognition* as a short research note. It was rejected as being too inconsequential. *Psychologia*, an obscure Japanese, English-language journal accepted it without revision, and it was published in 1987. In the ensuing 22 years, it has been cited twice. I am delighted that you, dear reader, now know the fuller story of this pilgrim's progress to understanding. Perhaps it will influence the way you do social psychology, in the lab and in your life . . .

> The artist, then, like the thinker or the scientist, seeks the truth and makes his appeal. Impressed by the aspect of the world, the thinker plunges into ideas, the scientist into facts—whence, presently emerging, they make their appeal to those qualities of our being that fit us best for the hazardous enterprise of living.
>
> Conrad, *Preface to The Nigger of the Narcissus*

REFERENCES

Bacon, F. (1620/2000). *The new organon* (edited by L. Jardine & M. Silverthorne). New York: Cambridge University Press.

Bond, M. H. (1972). The effect of an impression set on subsequent behavior. *Journal of Personality and Social Psychology, 24*, 301–305.

Bond, M. H. (1987). Old wine in new skins: Impressions about others can be disconfirmed by social reality! *Psychologia, 30*, 39–43.

Mischel, W. (1968). *Personality and assessment*. New York: Wiley.

Rosenthal, R., & Jacobson, L. (1968). *Pygmalion in the classroom: Teacher expectation and pupils' intellectual development.* New York: Holt, Rinehart, and Winston.

Snyder, M., & Stukas, A. A., Jr. (1999). Interpersonal processes: The interplay of cognitive, motivational, and behavioral activities in social interaction. *Annual Review of Psychology, 50,* 273–303.

DAN BATSON, University of Kansas

Bet You Didn't Know I Did a Dissonance Study

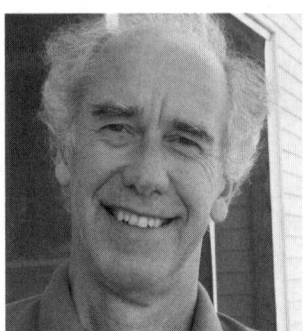

In the invitation to write this brief self-disclosure, Bob Arkin described the consistent response of visitors to Ohio State when he asked what they thought was their most underappreciated work: first, a blank "start," then a faint smile, a look into the middle distance, and, within about 15 seconds, the start of a story about a mistreated product. Thinking about Bob's question, I went through roughly the same sequence. My faint smile was at realizing that my most underappreciated work changes, and predictably. It is the work for which I have just read the action letter and reviews. I also realized that this judgment about lack of appreciation is deeply clouded and, in retrospect, almost always wrong. For a less biased and more justified assessment, it seemed wise to apply something like the historian's rule of not judging anything less than 50 years old. Having no work of that vintage, I had to substitute 30 for 50. The attempt to see back 30 years produced my look into the middle distance. And although it took a little longer than 15 seconds for a story to come to mind, one did. Here it is—as best I remember it.

When taking a course in Psychology of Religion at Princeton Theological Seminary in the spring of 1966, I was casting about for a topic for the term paper. The instructor's orientation was psychodynamic, but he said we could attempt an empirical project if we dared. Somewhere I had picked up a copy of *When Prophecy Fails* by Festinger, Riecken, and Schachter (1956), complete with Mrs. Keech, the Seekers, messages from Planet Clarion, prediction of flood and rescue, failure of the flying saucer to appear on that cold December night, and the subsequent increase in fervor and proselytizing by the faithful. On the first page of Chapter 1, Festinger et al. (1956) claimed the process they observed was not unique to the Seekers:

> Man's resourcefulness goes beyond simply protecting a belief. Suppose an individual believes something with his whole heart; suppose further that he has a commitment to this belief, that he has taken irrevocable actions because of it; finally, suppose that he is presented with evidence, unequivocal and undeniable evidence, that his belief is wrong: what will happen? The individual will frequently emerge, not only unshaken, but even more convinced of the truth of his beliefs than ever before. Indeed, he may even show a new fervor about convincing and converting other people to his view. (p. 3)

It was hard to miss the possible parallel to events surrounding the origins of Christianity, and Festinger et al.—delicately—made sure the reader did not. I thought: Is it really true that if you provide professed Christians with clear evidence that Christianity is a hoax, they will respond by affirming their belief even more strongly? Might make a term paper. So I set about designing a study.

Necessary ingredients were (a) professed Christians and (b) disconfirming information—clear evidence that Christianity is a hoax. Not having totally "unequivocal and undeniable evidence," I looked for professed Christians who might believe what evidence I could provide. Several friends at the seminary worked with church youth programs, and they agreed to integrate my study into their programs as a means to stimulate thought and discussion about the nature of religious beliefs and reactions to contrary evidence.

Participants for the study were 50 female high-school students. (I was concerned that males attending the programs might be there for the females, not the religion.) As they entered the room being used for the research, participants were asked to sit in one of two distinct locations, depending on whether they answered yes or no to the question: "Do you believe Jesus is the Son of God?" For the 42 participants who said yes, this produced public commitment and action—conditions specified by Festinger et al. (1956) as necessary to get belief intensification in the face of disconfirming information. Once seated, participants were given a booklet that contained, first, a 30-item questionnaire to measure strength of initial belief in the divinity of Jesus and the infallibility of the Bible (the 30 items were randomly chosen from a pool of 50). Next came an article "written anonymously and denied publication in the *New York Times* because of the obvious crushing effect if would have on the entire Christian world," followed by a second questionnaire with the 20 remaining belief items and, consistent with the cover story about testing reactions to the article and whether it should be published, 12 items about the article.

The article was my source of disconfirming information. It began:

—Geneva, Switzerland. It was learned today here in Geneva from a top source in the World Council of Churches offices that scholars in Jordan have conclusively proved that the major writings in what is today called the New Testament are fraudulent.

The article went on to describe the recent discovery of papyrus scrolls in the desert near where the Dead Sea Scrolls had been found. The scrolls included letters between the composers of various New Testament books. One bluntly stated:

"Since our great teacher Jesus of Nazareth was killed by the Romans, I am sure we were justified in stealing away his body and claiming that he rose from the dead. For, although his death clearly proves he was not the Son of God as we had hoped, if we did not claim that he was, both his great teaching and our lives as his disciples would be wasted."

The article then quoted modern church authorities, who admitted that "radiocarbon dating and careful study of the Aramaic dialect" unequivocally established the authenticity of the scrolls, yet insisted, "We just can't let this story get out!" It ended:

Apparently, the only avenue open to the Church in the twentieth century is the same avenue which it took in the first century—conceal the facts and proclaim Jesus as the divine Son of God, even though it knows such a claim is a lie.

My fears that no one would believe the article was true were somewhat allayed when I went to pick up copies of the booklet from the duplicating center at the seminary. The student working there was wide-eyed when I came in: "Where did you get this; is it really true?!" If the article caused a seminarian to doubt, at least some high-school students might be fooled.

As it turned out, some participants did believe the article was true; some did not. Consistent with the claims of Festinger et al. (1956), participants who both (a) publicly self-identified as believing Jesus was the Son of God and (b) said they believed the article was true had significantly higher belief scores on the posttest than the pretest. Belief scores dropped for other participants. I reported the study in my term paper, noting the support for dissonance theory, and moved on to other things.

ITS IMPACT

After four more years at the seminary, graduate school in psychology, and a move to Kansas, I had the chance to sit in on a graduate seminar taught by Mike Storms.

One week, Mike was pushing a cool-information-processing/self-perception interpretation of dissonance research. I tried to think of dissonance effects that could not be accounted for in this way, and the study I did in seminary came to mind. Looking back, the results seemed impossible to explain in terms of cool, rational processing. So I wrote up the study under the title "Rational processing or rationalization? The effect of disconfirming information on a stated religious belief." I showed the write-up to Mike and, encouraged by him, sent it off to *JPSP*. It received a quite positive review (only one review, as I recall) and an action letter of acceptance pending minor revision. Enclosed with the action letter, which was sent from Hawaii, was a pressed orchid—a delightful editorial touch!

The paper was published in *JPSP* in 1975 and, thereafter, almost entirely ignored—well, at least until recently. PsycInfo says it has been cited 31 times, 27 of these since 1997. (I believe Eddie Harmon-Jones is primarily responsible for the late surge.) Why was the paper ignored? Several possible reasons come to mind.

First, the study did not fit within the orthodox lines of dissonance research; it was not an induced-compliance, free-choice, or even selective-exposure study. Belief intensification in the face of disconfirming information has often been overlooked as a dissonance phenomenon despite the early attention it received from Festinger et al. (1956). This is a shame because it really does seem to be a clear, direct prediction of the theory, one with wide-ranging and important implications—for scientific believers as well as religious ones—that cannot be explained by competing theories.

Second, the word "dissonance" did not appear in the title of the paper. Authors of a major review of the dissonance literature completed the year following publication of the paper missed it, I was told, as a result. Failure to recognize that the paper was about dissonance would be less likely today; the first two words of the abstract, "cognitive dissonance," would be picked up as keywords in a database search. Still, the moral of this part of the story is: Talk in categories in play in the field, using terminology and titles that pigeonhole you properly. (If possible, however, resist having your thinking constrained by these categories.) Interestingly, "dissonance" also did not appear in the Festinger et al. (1956) title or even in their index; instead, "consonance-dissonance theory" was in the index. Could this be one reason *When Prophecy Fails* is often omitted from the dissonance canon?

Third, the procedure of the study was admittedly complex, audacious, potentially offensive, and ethically questionable. Likely, neither the procedure I used nor any similar one could be run today. There were no sequels, spin-offs, or rebuttals.

Finally, the year before the paper was published, Zanna and Cooper (1974) provided their elegant demonstration that dissonance was not a cool process, using a misattribution manipulation in an induced-compliance paradigm. Their study was very much in the mainstream of the discipline and gained immediate and well-deserved attention. My oddball study was ignored.

UNDERAPPRECIATED?

Am I bitter about the reception my study received? Not bitter, but perhaps a little wistful. On the one hand, it was my first try at psychological research, conceived and conducted with embarrassing ignorance of the relevant literature. Having simply stumbled on a little-recognized but important dissonance process, I look at the study as a bit of underappreciated serendipity. On the other hand, I think I got an *A* on my term paper for the Psychology of Religion class. And the psychological research I worked on next, also serendipitous, is probably my most over-appreciated and got me on a wave I've been riding ever since—the Good Samaritan study done with John Darley (Darley & Batson, 1973). Maybe it all evens out.

REFERENCES

Batson, C. D. (1975). Rational processing or rationalization? The effect of disconfirming information on a stated religious belief. *Journal of Personality and Social Psychology, 32,* 176–184.

Darley, J. M., & Batson, C. D. (1973). "From Jerusalem to Jericho": A study of situational and dispositional variables in helping behavior. *Journal of Personality and Social Psychology, 27,* 100–108.

Festinger, L., Riecken, H. W., & Schachter, S. (1956). *When prophecy fails: A social and psychological study of a modern group that predicted the destruction of the world.* Minneapolis: University of Minnesota Press.

Zanna, M. P., & Cooper, J. (1974). Dissonance and the pill: An attribution approach to studying the arousal properties of dissonance. *Journal of Personality and Social Psychology, 29,* 703–709.

JERRY M. BURGER, Santa Clara University

Is That All There Is? Reaction to the That's-Not-All Procedure

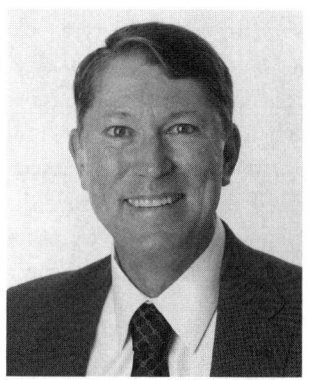

Many years ago, I published a set of seven studies on a compliance tactic I dubbed the "that's-not-all" technique (Burger, 1986). Like the foot-in-the-door, the door-in-the-face, and the low-ball that preceded it, the "that's-not-all" procedure is a sequential-request tactic—that is, the requester sets up the targeted individual with one request, which leads to an increased likelihood of compliance to a second request. Briefly, someone using the tactic presents a request at a certain price, makes the individual ponder the offer rather than allowing him or her to respond, and then sweetens the deal. The improved offer often comes in the form of an added benefit (e.g., free shipping) or a lower price. If the technique works, people are more likely to comply with the request than if they had been presented with the improved offer at the outset.

THE INSPIRATION AND THE PROCESS

The studies were inspired in part by an approach to social influence research advocated by Robert Cialdini (1980). Cialdini argues that researchers would do well to open their eyes to what professional influencers are doing all around them. Salespeople, recruiters, and the like have spent years developing tactics to get potential customers and volunteers to say "yes." Thus, step one in the process is what Cialdini calls "systematic personal observation." Watch what the pros do; their livelihood depends on figuring out ways to increase compliance. Step two is to find out if the tactic you've observed really works. Professional salespeople, after all, could also be fooled by illusory correlations. Next, demonstrate the effect using the empirical tools of our trade. Better yet, replicate the effect using different procedures and different populations. The third step is the hardest. Explain why the tactic increases compliance. Identify the psychological processes underlying the effect and produce evidence in support of that explanation. If everything works as it is supposed to, you'll end up with a package of studies demonstrating an interesting social influence phenomenon with obvious real-world applications.

Step one for me—the observation—took place when my wife and I were looking into buying a membership at a local gym. After showing us around, the manager wrote the cost of a year's membership for two on a piece of paper and set the paper on the desk in front of me. He then distracted himself with something-or-other for a few seconds, which allowed me to ponder the figure on the paper before me. Next, no doubt after counting to a certain number in his head, the manager turned the paper over and wrote a substantially lower price that he was prepared to offer me for the membership. I could feel the pull of the persuasion; I was almost ready to buy a new gym bag.

Step two—demonstrating the effect—started with two field investigations. In both studies, we set up bake sale tables at various locations in the community and on campus. We had plenty of cupcakes on display, but no indication of prices anywhere. In Study 1, when people approached the table and asked one of the two experimenters the price, those assigned to the experimental condition were told the cupcakes were 75 cents each. At that precise moment, the second experimenter interrupted, and the first experimenter held up an open palm to prevent a response. After a few seconds, the first experimenter lowered his or her hand and explained that the price also included a bag of cookies, which suddenly appeared from somewhere under the table. That procedure led to a significantly higher rate of compliance than when participants were simply shown the cookies and told the cupcake-and-cookie package was 75 cents. In Study 2, lowering the price from $1.00 to 75 cents while the participants stared at the open palm also increased sales over a condition in which the experimenter simply gave the 75-cent price. That's-not-all appeared to work.

I began the third step by identifying two processes I thought might be responsible for the effect. One of these was the norm of reciprocity. According to this social rule, people feel a need to return favors. Participants in our studies might have interpreted the improved offer as a type of favor from the experimenter, which they could reciprocate by buying the cupcake. The second explanation was taken from Sherif's social judgment theory. When making a judgment, such as whether

75 cents for a cupcake is a good deal, people rely on some kind of anchor point. By giving the initial price as $1.00, the experimenter may have suggested an anchor point that the participant then used when making this judgment. When compared against a $1.00 anchor point, 75 cents seems like a reasonable price. Studies 3, 4, and 5 found evidence for both of these explanations. Study 6 ruled out an alternate explanation based a simple contrast effect, and Study 7 demonstrated how that's-not-all was different from the door-in-the-face procedure.

In short, I thought I had done everything right. I had conducted seven experiments, some in the field and some in the lab. I had demonstrated the robustness of the effect using different methodologies and different participants. I had examined the psychological processes underlying the effect and presented evidence in support of my explanations. And, following the tradition established by those before me, I had given this new compliance tactic an eye-grabbing and slightly whimsical name. I published the paper in the *Journal of Personality and Social Psychology*, the most visible journal in the field. Certainly a tidal wave of that's-not-all studies was on the horizon.

HARDLY A RIPPLE

It's been more than two decades since I published the original paper. In that time, I am aware of only two other articles that report research on that's-not-all—and one of those articles is mine. The other was published by Eric Knowles and some of his students in 1998. As far as I know, that's it. I imagine I would be first in line to serve as a reviewer should a that's-not-all paper fall into an editor's lap, yet I can remember reviewing only one other manuscript with a that's-not-all study, and that was for a regional communication journal. In fairness, that's-not-all has appeared in quite a few social psychology textbooks. And the original article has been cited a few dozen times. Anthony Pratkanis (2007) included the procedure on his list of 107 social influence tactics that have been studied experimentally. And I even found a description of the procedure once when thumbing through one of those "for dummies" volumes while killing time in a bookstore. But it's not exactly the foot-in-the-door procedure, for which I once found more than a hundred published studies.

Why hasn't there been more research on that's-not-all? I have a couple of hunches. First, the original article framed the research almost exclusively in terms of compliance—that is, here's another tactic you can use to get people to say yes. That might be the right approach for a marketing journal. But were I to do it over again, I would place much more emphasis on the underlying psychological processes and the broader implications of the research. Specifically, I would focus on the importance of anchor points, the ease with which they can be manipulated, and the many implications the research has for social influence and attitude change. Second, staying in do-it-over mode, I would drop the whole reciprocity idea and interpretation. I no longer think the norm of reciprocity has much if anything to do with the that's-not-all effect. But because that was the explanation I presented first, it appears to be the one most people remember. Textbooks typically lump that's-not-all in with other reciprocity-based effects, which makes the procedure look like just another example of the reciprocity norm. Of course, I am pleased to see the work cited anywhere, but mis-cited and misconstrued references fall short of what I once expected for this article.

I still think the article is a solid piece of scholarship. And I believe Cialdini's systematic observation method is an excellent way for researchers to discover effective social influence phenomena. If there's a lesson in all this, it probably has something to do with the presentation and the way the work is framed. Making a splash no doubt requires a good idea and some well-crafted research, but there's also something to be said for how you tell the story.

REFERENCES

Burger, J. M. (1986). Increasing compliance by improving the deal: The that's–not–all technique. *Journal of Personality and Social Psychology, 51,* 277–283.

Cialdini, R. B. (1980). Full-cycle social psychology. *Applied Social Psychology Annual, 1,* 21–45.

Pratkanis, A. R. (2007). Social influence analysis: An index of tactics. In A. R. Pratkanis (Ed.), *The science of social influence: Advances and future progress* (pp. 17–82). New York: Psychology Press.

CHARLES S. CARVER, University of Miami

My Brief Career in Modeling

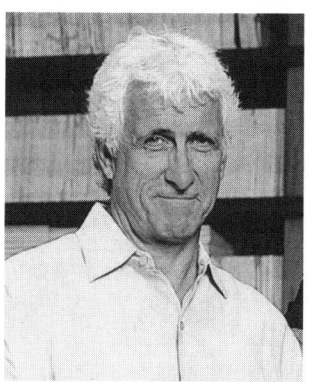

Early in my career I took up an idea from cognitive psychology about the coding of concept-related information and the coding of behavior-specifying information in memory. It was not a terribly profound idea: merely that these things were linked up somehow, such that recognizing something (activating the corresponding interpretive schema) also partially activated information pertaining to related action. (This was well before anyone had found mirror neurons, by the way.) Maybe the two sorts of information were part of a single schema, or maybe it was two schemas closely linked to one another (Schank & Abelson, 1977). In either case, it seemed reasonable to suggest that activating the interpretive information would render the behavioral information more accessible. This was a time when schemas for construal were being vigorously discussed, but not so many people were discussing the influence of construal on action (an exception was Wilson & Capitman [1982]).

At the same time I had been teaching introductory psychology on a regular basis. I had always been a little uncertain what to say regarding the group of modeling effects in which watching someone do something tends to induce the observer to do the same thing. These were typically called "releasing" or "response facilitation" effects—today they are sometimes called mimicry. They aren't observational learning (the behavior isn't new) and they do not obviously involve vicarious reinforcement (no one is being rewarded for anything)—it's just "person see, person do." Interpretations of these effects tended to allude vaguely to implicit reinforcers, but that had never seemed very satisfying to me. It dawned on me at some point that these effects might reflect close links in memory between information used for construal and information specifying how-to-do-it. These effects might well be a sort of accessibility effect.

Three colleagues and I (Carver, Ganellen, Froming, & Chambers, 1983) set out to test the plausibility of this reasoning. We took inspiration (and procedures) from a literature showing that activating a given informational category in memory makes that category more likely to be used later on, even in an unrelated context. Our chain of reasoning had two links. The first link is that seeing a model act in a particular way activates an interpretive schema; such an activation would be reflected in the use of the schema later if an opportunity to do so occurs. The second link is that activating an interpretive schema activates relevant behavioral information; such activation would be reflected if the quality in the schema were displayed in the person's behavior later.

These two links were tested in two experiments. In one experiment, subjects (they were subjects, back then) first watched a videotape portraying an interaction between a man and his secretary. The man either behaved neutrally or expressed overt annoyance and hostility toward the secretary. In an ostensibly unrelated second procedure, the subjects then completed a person-perception task. They read a description that had been constructed to be ambiguous with respect to the aggressiveness of the target person. Then they made ratings of the person. As predicted, observing an aggressive model caused subjects to perceive greater hostility in the ambiguous target person.

In a second experiment, we primed subjects' interpretive schemas with a sentence formation task that forced them to read (and therefore process) either a substantial number of words pertaining to aggression or only a few words pertaining to aggression. Then they engaged in a procedure in which they taught a concept to someone else via rewards and punishments, a common paradigm for studying aggression in terms of punishment intensities. In order to keep the prime from fading over time and events, training for the teaching task came first, then the prime, then the teaching task. To prevent subjects from realizing that the prime was relevant to the other task, the prime was administered by a second experimenter who said her subjects had not been showing up and begged the first experimenter to let the subject complete her brief measure. As predicted, priming aggressive verbal content led to more intense punishment.

So we had supported the links in our chain. So what? Modeling is a rather limited subset of the realm of human behavior. The broader implication of this work was that it gave credence to an information-processing account of how behavioral qualities emerge in the stream of behavior. This was a period in which the 25-year dominance of the learning-theory view of behavior was beginning to give way to the "cognitive revolution," and the evidence derived from this research was a small cannon shot in that revolution. A very small one. The manuscript was rejected by an associate editor at the *Journal of Personality and Social Psychology* because it did not take into account the Berkowitz neo-associationist theory of aggression (ahem, the paper was about modeling, not aggression). It eventually was published in another journal, whereupon it sank like a stone in a pond (though Len Berkowitz immediately cited it, approvingly).

In the course of writing this saga of underappreciation, I was somewhat surprised to discover that the paper seems to have been rescued from its obscurity in late life. John Bargh, who had developed his own extensive program of work on the priming of behavior, discovered and cited it, thereby inducing others to do so as well. After the article received favorable play in Bargh, Chen, and Burrows (1996), its citation rate tripled. This just goes to show that you never really know what's going to happen.

What advice does this experience lead me to offer new investigators? Now that I am no longer editing a journal, I would say it leads me to advise them to argue with editorial decisions. More seriously, I would advise people not to expect the importance of their work to be noticed immediately, but rather to view any case in which it does happen as being a delightful bonus. I think it may also be important to keep in play, in subsequent writing, any idea you think is being underappreciated, so that people have the opportunity to be exposed to it more than once. It sometimes takes more than one exposure to realize that something is interesting.

As for the impact of this research on my own future agenda, there was pretty much no impact at all. The pair of studies did what I had wanted to do: supported the idea that there is a close link from schemas for construal to schemas for action. I had satisfied myself that releasing effects have nothing to do with reinforcement. I moved on to other questions, many of them related to the same basic world view as had prompted these studies. But that was the end of my brief career in modeling.

REFERENCES

Bargh, J. A., Chen, M., & Burrows, L. (1996). Automaticity of social behavior: Direct effects of trait construct and stereotype activation on action. *Journal of Personality and Social Psychology, 71*, 230–244.

Carver, C. S., Ganellen, R. J., Froming, W. J., & Chambers, W. (1983). Modeling: An analysis in terms of category accessibility. *Journal of Experimental Social Psychology, 19*, 403–421.

Schank, R. C., & Abelson, R. P. (1977). *Scripts, plans, goals, and understanding.* Hillsdale, NJ: Erlbaum.

Wilson, T. D., & Capitman, J. A. (1982). Effects of script availability on social behavior. *Personality and Social Psychology Bulletin, 8*, 11–19.

GEORGE R. GOETHALS, University of Richmond

The Diversity of Social Support and Outgroup Homogeneity: Some Bad Luck and a Lot of Good Fortune

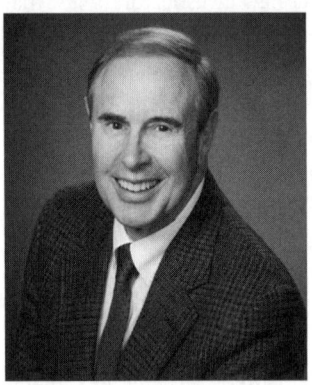

When Bob Arkin invited me to participate in this project, I knew immediately what I might write about, but the whole idea seemed quite freighted. It moves us, I think, toward ruminating self-servingly and writing bleatingly. I've found it a little easier to do that than I'd like to admit. Nevertheless, I am pleased to be included and to submit a contribution.

One reason that it feels strange to write for this collection is that I feel incredibly lucky in almost everything that has happened in my career. I have had more than my share of breaks, so encountering a little underappreciation along the way seems more than fair. On the side of good fortune, I was lucky enough to work with Ken Gergen as an undergraduate, and to follow his gentle guidance toward Duke for graduate school. There good things continued to happen, as I profited greatly from working primarily with Ned Jones, but also with Jack Brehm and Darwyn Linder. My interest in teaching took me to Williams College, where I was lucky enough to work for 36 years. During many of those years I collaborated with Williams colleagues Saul Kassin and Steve Fein. And during those years I had a number of valuable sabbaticals. An early one at Princeton re-established my working relationship with Joel Cooper from graduate school, and led to collaborations with John Darley and Mark Zanna. Later at the University of Virginia, Steve Worchel and I initiated a number of projects. A few years after that I had a leave at Santa Barbara, where I enjoyed working with Scott Allison, Dave Hamilton, Diane Mackie, and Dave Messick. Good and lasting friendships grew out of all of those collaborations.

My biggest breaks were that two of my publications in the 1970s got a fair amount of attention, thanks to colleagues. The first was my paper with Rick Reckman, a Williams undergraduate, called "The perception of consistency in attitudes." This paper showed how much individual attitudes, in this case toward school bussing, could be changed in a group, and how completely the participants, recent high school graduates, misremembered their initial attitudes. Though this paper, as noted at the time, was really just a replication of an earlier study published by Bem and McConnell, it received favorable attention in influential papers by Dick Nisbett and Tim Wilson and by Tony Greenwald. The second was the paper I co-authored with John Darley on an attributional analysis of social comparison. It articulated, though not really for the first time, an approach that Ladd Wheeler and Miron Zuckerman subsequently dubbed the "related attributes hypothesis." The naming may have been more important than the original idea, and led to the paper receiving lots of attention. Again, I was very fortunate.

So, what's not to like about the appreciation my work has received in the discipline? Well, there is one paper that perhaps could have been more noticed than it has been. In 1979, thanks to a lot of help from Bob Wyer (those of you who are now middle-aged, or older, surely all remember those multi-page, single-spaced reviews), *JESP* published an article that I co-authored with Shelley Allison and Marnie Frost. It was called "Perceptions of the magnitude and diversity of social support." It showed two things. First, people overestimate how many other people agree with them. This was not news, since Lee Ross had recently explored the false consensus effect. Second, and more important, people tend to see their own group—that is, the people who agree with them—as more diverse than those who disagree with them. Individuals like to believe that their views are not biased by personal characteristics, and that lots of different people share them. At the same time, they'd like to think that people on the other side of the fence are narrow, and probably biased. We showed this in three studies and argued that the phenomenon was widespread. For example, our paper noted that a group on our campus had described itself in the first sentence of its recruiting message as "a diverse group of students. . . ." Related to these results, at about the same time I presented an EPA paper in New York (Thane Pittman was the session chair) on people's varying perceptions of who fits what stereotypes. Republicans thought most Democrats fit the description we wrote of Democrats, but that fewer Republicans fit the description we wrote of Republicans. Democrats thought just the opposite. Stereotypes fit the outgroup, but not the ingroup. I liked that study, but like most EPA papers, this one sank out of sight.

At about the same time, Mick Rothbart and others explored what they called the "outgroup homogeneity effect." I remember thinking, why hadn't I coined that term? It was even better than the "related attributes hypothesis." Their work caused quite a stir, and I felt left on the sidelines. Hadn't I already shown perceptions of outgroup homogeneity, as well as ingroup diversity? Brian Mullen, bless his soul, always cited Goethals, Allison, and Frost (1979) when he published papers touching on outgroup homogeneity, but I think he was the only one.

In retrospect, I might have done two things differently. First, I might have been smart enough to realize that people's perceptions of outgroups are at least as important, probably more so, than their perceptions of ingroups. It would have been better to focus on that. Second, I should have remembered the importance of choosing a good title or label for certain findings. Ned Jones called my result showing that our confidence that we're correct is often more influenced by dissimilar agreers than similar agreers the "triangulation effect." That helped people notice a bit more than they might have otherwise. Later, Scott Allison, Dave Messick, and I published a paper showing people rate themselves as better than others on creativity, athleticism, fairness, and morality, but not on intelligence. We called our finding the "Muhammad Ali effect." This came from The Champ's answer to a question about whether he had deliberately faked a poor performance on the Army mental test to stay out of the service. He smiled and answered, "I said I was the greatest, not the smartest." That label actually took hold, and made the finding more visible. Perhaps if I had come up with a tag as good as the "outgroup homogeneity effect" my studies on perceptions of ingroup and outgroup diversity would have been more visible.

In short, the Goethals, Allison, and Frost paper is, for me, the most underappreciated. Anyway, that was some 30 years ago. Since then, my career and my life have had much more good fortune than bad. Things have balanced out very positively.

As I said before, I am very pleased to be included in this volume. I've been largely away from mainstream social psychology for some time. Starting in 1981, I got increasingly drawn into administration at Williams. By the time I finished a five-year stint as Provost in 1995, I had been more out of the field than in it—for over a decade. I then spent a wonderful leave at the University of Massachusetts, and sat in on Susan Fiske's excellent social cognition seminar. But my interests had evolved and it was too late to go back. I turned to some longstanding interests in history and politics, and taught a course on leadership. That led to an interdepartmental "concentration" in Leadership Studies at Williams, and my introduction to the Jepson School of Leadership Studies at the University of Richmond. In 2005 I was offered a professorship here, and I decided to leave Williams for Richmond. I have four wonderful social psychology colleagues at Richmond, Don Forsyth and Crystal Hoyt in the Jepson School, and Jeni Burnette and my former collaborator Scott Allison in the Psychology Department. Scott and I have resumed working together, on a number of topics. We have collaborated on a recent book about heroes, published, like the current volume, by Oxford. At the same time, I have begun doing history, of a kind, and have published a few papers on Ulysses S. Grant's military career and presidency, and will soon undertake a large project on how U.S. presidential leadership, from Washington to Obama, has advanced or retarded the rights and status of African Americans.

As I look back 40 years post-PhD, I have some thoughts that may be useful to younger generations of social psychologists. My career has been unusual, so it might not have any implications for most early career scholars. Nevertheless, I would offer the following. For many of us, life is long. It pays to be broad, to pay attention to what's going on in the world, inside and outside of academia. Keep alive and well your scholarly interests beyond psychology and beyond your narrower interests within psychology. I started college thinking I would be a history major. In some ways, my interest in leadership studies combines my more formal work in psychology with my informal interests in history. It's all come together. Reading history along the way has been fun and, ultimately, useful. Stay broad.

Second, stay connected. As noted, I have benefited enormously from collaborations of various kinds with other social psychologists at other places, mostly large research universities. This is especially important if you go the liberal arts college route. If you can, make sure your school has a good leave policy, and take the word "leave" literally. Go, and return, when you can. That's harder now than a generation ago, with labs that need looking after and dual careers. But it very much helps staying broad and staying connected.

Third, stay up to date. That's also getting harder, especially if you get diverted into things like administration. But it is critical. You don't want to find yourself beached at age 50 or 60 or even 70 having lost contact with your scholarly field. In that regard, think carefully about the pros and cons of taking on chair or dean roles. They can be very challenging and very satisfying, but they work against the three suggestions above.

Finally, I would encourage you to think carefully about what is really important and interesting, outside your specialty as well as in it. Will anybody care? What chances does your work have of finding its way into a social psychology textbook, and perhaps reaching and teaching a broader audience? Does it shed important light on interesting psychological questions or phenomena? Back to my own example of "most underappreciated," part of this is framing, or, less charitably, packaging. Concepts such as the outgroup homogeneity effect and the hindsight bias capture and point to something important. Labels such as "perceptions of the magnitude and diversity of social support" can miss badly. Consider how you can best generate interest in your work. One hint. At a wedding, an undergraduate mentor, anthropologist John Whiting, asked me what my PhD dissertation was about. I told him it was complicated. He said it should be a requirement of the PhD to be able to summarize your thesis in one sentence. That was good advice: What's the take-home message?

I hope that some of these observations are useful to some readers in thinking about structuring their lives and careers. They may be too idiosyncratic. For me they have much do with the fact that professional life continues to be fortunate and fulfilling. I haven't been underappreciated.

REFERENCES

Allison, S. T., & Goethals, G.R. (in press). *Heroes, what they do & why we need them*. New York: Oxford University Press.

Allison, S. T., Messick, D. M., & Goethals, G. R. (1989). On being better but not smarter than others: The Muhammad Ali effect. *Social Cognition, 7*, 275–295.

Goethals, G. R., Allison, S. J., & Frost, M. (1979). Perceptions of the magnitude and diversity of social support. *Journal of Experimental Social Psychology, 15*, 570–581.

Goethals, G. R., & Darley, J. M. (1977). Social comparison theory: An attributional approach. In J. M. Suls, & R. L. Miller, (Eds.), *Social comparisons processes: Theoretical and empirical perspectives*. Washington, DC: Hemisphere Publishing Corporation.

LADD WHEELER, Macquarie University, Sydney, Australia

Thirty Years of Contrast in Social Comparison

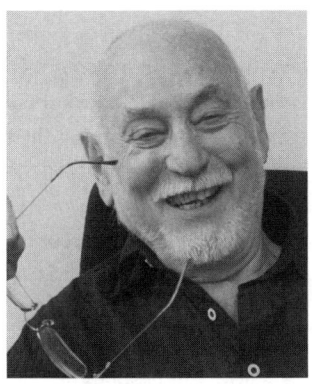

My advisor in graduate school was Stan Schachter,[1] who taught a year-long seminar at the University of Minnesota on social comparison theory and its antecedents. Stan had been involved in the work that led up to social comparison theory and knew why every step had been taken. Under his masterful guidance, we explored these steps one by one and tried to predict what would happen next. All the social psychology graduate students took the seminar, as well as many from outside social. It was an extraordinarily stimulating and competitive year. The heart of social comparison theory (Festinger, 1954) was that people compare with those who are similar to them in order to evaluate themselves, and in the case of abilities, there is a unidirectional drive upward—so people want to be better than others, but not a lot better. It was not entirely clear whether the unidirectional drive should always lead to upward comparison, and the prospect of downward comparisons as well as upward comparisons was a topic of conversation in that remarkable seminar. After all, if people have a drive to be better than others, they might satisfy that drive by comparing with those who are *less* able than they are. There was no direct evidence about any of this because no research had given participants a choice between upward and downward comparison with people of varying levels of similarity to the participant.

To accomplish this, I devised what came to be known as the "rank-order paradigm." Participants were given their score on a bogus but positive personality test called "intellectual flexibility" and were told that they ranked fourth in their tested group of seven. Then, they were told that they could see the score of one other person in the group, and the rank of the person whose score they chose to see was the major dependent variable. I also manipulated the strength of the motivation to do well on the test. Finally, in order to tie the choice to the notion of similarity, I asked participants to indicate which person they thought they were most similar to in score. The answer of course had to be the person at rank 5 or at rank 3.

I found that participants compared with the most similar person in the upward direction (rank 3), particularly when they were more motivated to do well. Not only did participants in general say that they were more similar to rank 3, but those who said this were the most likely to choose to see the score at rank 3. I interpreted this as indicating that participants assumed similarity with the person above them in the rank order and then chose to see that score in the hope of confirming their similarity. I concluded that upward comparison is used to confirm that one is "almost as good as the very good ones" (Wheeler, 1966, p. 30).

The research was published in 1966, a long version having been rejected a couple of times, in the first and only supplement to the *Journal of Experimental Social Psychology*, under special editor Bibb Latané, one of my fellow graduate students and friend to regular editor John Thibaut. This collection contained two other experiments using the rank-order paradigm done by fellow Minnesota graduate students after the completion of my research. Karl Hakmiller in his dissertation research showed that downward comparison occurred when participants scored unexpectedly high on an undesirable personality trait. John Arrowood (with student Dorothy Thornton), at the University of Toronto after leaving Minnesota, showed that a positive instance of a trait was apparently more important than similarity on that trait. From then on, for the next decade or so, rank- order paradigm studies attempted to define the set of variables determining upward/downward choice as well as another twist, the selection of extreme scores (to explore the range of things) versus similar scores (to center in on one's own status). The finding from my dissertation, that people assume upward similarity and that this appears to mediate upward comparison choice, got completely lost in the flurry. It wasn't until Rebecca Collins (1996) published her paper on upward assimilation theory that my finding, now three decades ripened on the vine, became important and got some recognition. Collins argued that if people expect, for whatever reason, to be similar to an upward comparison target, they are more likely to construe differences as negligible and to assimilate to the target, with a positive change in self-evaluation. Current theories, such as Mussweiler's Selective Accessibility Model (2003), argue that the hypothesis of similarity with a target is the default hypothesis that people attempt to confirm and, in so doing, make accessible information consistent with the hypothesis (leading to assimilation). So if people initially perceive a global similarity with someone who is better, they tend to access other aspects that allow them to identify or assimilate in an upward direction. This should be no surprise, as the pre-eminence of the enhancement motive in the self-system is now fairly well established (e.g., Sedikides, 1993).

For 30 years between my dissertation and Collins's upward assimilation paper, most people thought that the default response to an upward comparison was contrast—as in the famous Mr. Clean/Mr. Dirty experiment by Morse and Gergen (1970). Now there is a great deal of interest in upward assimilation—so much that Jerry Suls and I have recently tried to bring some order to the area by discussing what assimilation is and what it isn't (Wheeler & Suls, 2007), and what is necessary to show it.

If there is a lesson to be learned from this experience, it is that one should not lose sight of one's discoveries when the rest of the world is proclaiming that other things are more important. As social psychologists, we ought to be fairly hip to social influence, but I wasn't in this case: I let the assimilation discovery get lost while I followed the MacGuffin.

NOTE

1. Schachter left Minnesota for Columbia in 1961, and Ben Willerman and Dana Bramel directed my dissertation. Dana, who was a new Festinger PhD from Stanford, even did double duty as my experimental confederate. I knew and admired Dana already from my undergraduate days at Stanford.

REFERENCES

Collins, R. L. (1996). For better or worse: The impact of upward social comparison on self-evaluations. *Psychological Bulletin, 119*, 51–69.

Festinger, L. (1954). A theory of social comparison processes. *Human Relations, 7*, 117–140.

Hakmiller, K. (1966). Threat as a determinant of downward comparison. *Journal of Experimental Social Psychology, 2*(Suppl. 1), 32–39.

Morse, S., & Gergen, K.J. (1970). Social comparison, self-consistency, and the concept of self. *Journal of Personality and Social Psychology, 16*, 148–156.

Mussweiler, T. (2003). Comparison processes in social judgment: Mechanisms and consequences. *Psychological Review, 110*(3), 472–489.

Sedikides, C. (1993). Assessment, enhancement, and verification determinants of the self-evaluation process. *Journal of Personality and Social Psychology, 65*, 317–338.

Thornton, D. A., & Arrowood, J. (1966). Self-evaluation, self-enhancement, and the locus of social comparison. *Journal of Experimental Social Psychology, 2*(Suppl. 1), 40–48.

Wheeler, L. (1966). Motivation as a determinant of upward comparison. *Journal of Experimental Social Psychology, 2*(Suppl. 1), 27–31.

Wheeler, L., & Suls, J. (2007). Assimilation in social comparison: Can we agree on what it is? *International Review of Social Psychology, 20*(1), 31–51.

CONSTANTINE SEDIKIDES, University of Southampton

The Causal Structure of Person Types and Stereotypes

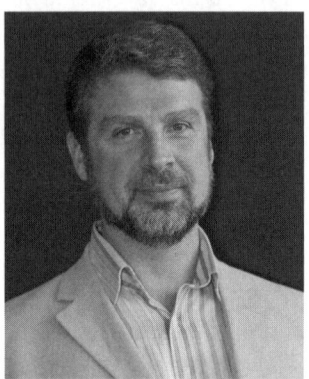

I can trace my interest in causality back to my undergraduate years, when I became acquainted with philosophical thinking on the topic. I was delighted when, as a first-year graduate student at the Ohio State University (OSU), I had the opportunity to work with Craig Anderson. Craig was spending the year (1984–85) visiting at the OSU, and he offered a stimulating graduate seminar on causal thinking covering in part his ongoing and fascinating research on knowledge structures. I could not believe my luck when Craig indicated that he was willing to work with me! The fruits of our joint research (Anderson & Sedikides, 1991; Sedikides & Anderson, 1992, 1994) on implicit personality theory were most rewarding for me, both professionally and personally. One of these fruits, however, the Sedikides and Anderson (1994) article, did not appear to be that sweet to my colleagues. In fact, it has been more forbidden than sweet.

This article capitalized on the so-called typological view of person perception (Anderson & Sedikides, 1991). People, this view has it, think about others' personalities in terms of types. A person type consists of several traits. For example, the type "depressed" consists of the traits *lonely, gloomy, pessimistic, unhappy,* and *fearful.* The type "intellectual" consists of the traits *intelligent, efficient, competent,* and *studious*. And the type "unsocialized" consists of the traits *rebellious, disobedient, inconsistent, careless,* and *lazy*. From a methodological standpoint, person types are operationalized as clusters. Cluster analysis establishes traits as members of a given type according to two criteria: how close traits are to each other, and how far traits are from other clusters.

Person types have interesting properties. Knowing one trait within a given type allows one to predict other traits in the same type. More importantly, traits within types have a rather mysterious form of interconnectedness. Traits hang out with each other. Is it because traits are seen as covarying or associated with each other, as indicated by Pearson product-moment correlation coefficients? For example, if one is seen as honest, one may also be seen as trustworthy. Alternatively, is it because traits are summarized in terms of global dimensions such as evaluation (i.e., positive/negative) or dynamism (i.e., strong/weak), as typically indicated by multidimensional scaling (MDS) analyses? Albeit plausible, these possibilities could not fully account for the data (Anderson & Sedikides, 1991). What is it, then, that keeps the traits together within a type? What sort of glue is this?

We (Sedikides & Anderson, 1994) reasoned that this glue is causal. Traits within each person type are seen as causing each other. Take, for instance, the type "depressed." Being *lonely* may cause someone to be *gloomy* and *pessimistic*, which in turn causes that person to be *unhappy* and subsequently *fearful*. Now, think of the type "intellectual." Being *intelligent* makes someone *studious*, which turns him or her into *efficient* and, in the long term, *competent*. Finally, consider the type "unsocialized." Being *lazy* leads someone to be *careless*, which causes that person to be *inconsistent*, which (perhaps in reactance to frequent negative feedback) makes him or her *disobedient* and, in the long run, *rebellious*. Such causal sequences made sense to us.

We put these ideas to the test. Before I describe the testing procedure, I will digress a little and define three constructs. A given person type includes both core and noncore trait members. *Core members* are those traits that are intercorrelated highly; that is, they are the strongest, or most prototypical, members of that person type. *Noncore members* are those traits that have the lowest intercorrelations with the other members; they are the weakest members of the type. Finally, I will need to define *strong nonmembers*. These are traits that do not belong to the person type in question (i.e., they are not cluster members) but nevertheless have two notable properties: They feature (a) higher average intercorrelations with the core members than the noncore members, and (b) smaller MDS distances from the core members than the noncore members. Despite these properties, strong nonmembers are intriguingly seen as a poorer fit with individual core members than are noncore members (Anderson & Sedikides, 1991).

Back to the testing of the idea that traits within each type are causally interconnected (Sedikides & Anderson, 1994, Experiment 1). For each person type, we derived all possible combinations of two kinds of trait pairs. The first kind of pair was core/noncore members (32 pairs in all). The second kind of pair was core members/strong nonmembers (150 pairs in all). Then, we asked participants to make causation ratings on those 182 pairs. In particular, for each trait pair, participants made the following judgment: how likely is it for the first trait in the pair to cause or underlie the second trait?

We proceeded with comparing the mean causation rating for core/noncore member pairs with the mean causation rating for core/strong nonmembers pairs. What would constitute support for the hypothesis that person types consist of causally linked traits? Simply, the average causation rating for core/noncore members trait pairs ought to be higher than the average causation rating for core/strong nonmembers trait pairs. There is a way to put it in English. Noncore members ought to be more causally related to the core members than are strong nonmembers, even though the latter are both more highly correlated with core members and closer in MDS space to core members. This is indeed what we found! The hypothesis that causal connections glue together traits within person types received empirical backing.

We tested the same hypothesis in a different way (Sedikides & Anderson, 1994, Experiment 2). We asked whether traits within a person type are seen as more causally related to one another than to other traits that share the *same* MDS space. We relied on three sets of closely related person types (from Anderson & Sedikides, 1991). For each set, participants rated how causally related they perceived the various trait pairs to be; that is, they judged how likely a trait was to cause or underlie another trait. They rated all possible pairs of traits within the relevant MDS space. Then, we compared average within-type ratings (pairs of traits from the same person type) with average between-type ratings (pairs of traits not from the same person type). The hypothesis was, once again, confirmed. Within-type members were seen as more causally linked to each other than to members of other types, even when all were located in the same MDS space.

The research has implications for understanding person perception and person memory. The research consolidated the finding that people perceive others in terms of person types. More to the point, the research provided insights into the internal structure of person types: traits within each type are causally connected. This has implications for the person memory literature, which is concerned with the processing of information that is consistent or inconsistent with a prior impression. A problem that has plagued this literature has to do with adequate conceptual and operational definitions of consistency or inconsistency. Our findings addressed this problem. A prior impression can be conceptualized as a trait in a given person type. If so, consistent traits are those with positive causal connections to this trait, whereas inconsistent traits are those with negative causal connections to this trait.

Our research also has implications for intergroup perception (i.e., stereotyping). Person types can be broadly conceived as a form of stereotypes. As such, our research alludes to the complex structure of stereotypes. Often, stereotypes are seen as incoherent or as having evaluatively opposite traits. From the perspective of our research, such stereotypes are not incoherent; rather, they have an orderly causal structure. In particular, the evaluatively opposite traits are linked causally. Such stereotypes may consist of a hierarchically arranged system of features, so that the superordinate feature (e.g., ethnicity, age, gender, occupation) is perceived as causally linked to two subordinate traits that are themselves seen as negatively linked. For example, the type "actor" may be causally linked to both *gregarious* and *self-absorbed*, even though these two traits are negatively linked with each other. Likewise, the type "old" may be causally linked to *wise* and *out of touch*, even though these two traits are negatively related to one another.

In addition, our research has implications for self-perception, and in particular self-complexity. One way in which this construct has been operationalized is by having participants sort a number of traits into groups according to which traits seem to belong together. What implicit rules do participants follow in the trait sorting task? Our findings suggests that they follow implicit causality rules. They toss traits in a pile on the basis of person types, according to the "glue" of causality. Here, however, it is possible that, strength of causal connections being equal, positive traits are favored more than negative traits, a hypothesis that awaits verification. In fact, with recent advances in the measurement of implicit cognitions, causal connections in self-types (and also person types and stereotypes) would be better understood.

Furthermore, our conceptualization of stereotypes as person types provides a compelling explanation for why stereotypes are resistant to change. Traits comprising stereotypes are causally interconnected, and causal connections are notoriously resistant to change. At the same time, our research gives some guidance on how to proceed with a stereotype change agenda. Persuasive communication about ethnic, age, gender, weight, or occupational stereotypes that focuses on causal thinking (e.g., challenging malicious causal links or fostering benign links) is likely to be more effective than comparable communication that focuses on non-causal thinking (e.g., moralizing).

Our article, at the time, appeared to our biased eyes as a textbook case of a "good" article. It addressed an important problem; relied on a solid rationale; offered a novel hypothesis that could account for longstanding controversies in the field; used elaborate methodology; produced hypothesis-confirming results; and promised to be generative, with implications relevant to both (basic and applied) research as well as real-world interventions. The article reflected a programmatic, theory-driven approach to research, and produced applicable findings. What happened, then?

Granted, the article has not been completely ignored. A Google search (September 2010) indicated that it has been cited 25 times. However, this little-engine-that-could has not exactly taken the field by storm. Why so, it is hard to tell. Perhaps because I did not follow it up and did not pursue the implications of these findings. The field (like any vibrant and diverse scholarly field) needs to hear a certain message again and again, and then once more, before it begins to assimilate it. Although these studies were part of programmatic research, they came at the tail end of it. Thus, a new wave of experimentation that would build on the latest findings and produce an extended body of work might have brought along better the idea. Perhaps the reason why the article was not terribly influential has to do with the methodology: It was rather involved and cumbersome. Or, perhaps the message was not pitched at the right tone or level of analysis for the intended audience. Or, perhaps the idea (horror of horrors) was not that revolutionary. And a contributing factor may be that subsequent research agendas did not prioritize causal social knowledge or stereotype structure. We shall never know.

Regardless, I felt I benefited a lot from this work. I appreciated better Craig Anderson's theoretical orientation and methodological sophistication; I satisfied my interest in causal structures through a grounded, empirical approach; I made renewed contact with the person memory and stereotyping literatures; and I familiarized myself better with interesting statistical techniques. Last but not least, I changed the way I think about cognitive structures. To me, a "proper" cognitive structure is a causal structure. Research may end up being relatively unappreciated from others (usually for good reasons), but not necessarily from the perspective of the researcher.

REFERENCES

Anderson, C. A., & Sedikides, C. (1991). Contributions of a typological approach to associationistic and dimensional views of person perception. *Journal of Personality and Social Psychology, 60,* 203–217.

Sedikides, C., & Anderson, C. A. (1992). Causal explanations of defection: A knowledge structure approach. *Personality and Social Psychology Bulletin, 18,* 420–429.

Sedikides, C., & Anderson, C. A. (1994). Causal perceptions of inter-trait relations: The glue that holds person types together. *Personality and Social Psychology Bulletin, 20,* 294–302.

DAVID A. SCHROEDER, University of Arkansas

Your First Word Will Be Your Last Word if It Is Your Only Word

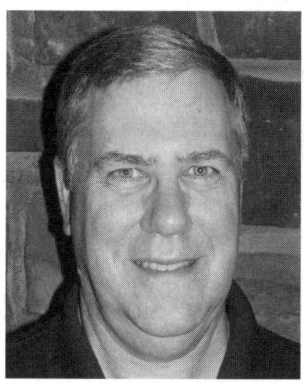

Many years ago, three (now former) students and I published an article entitled, "Attributions and attribution-relations: The effect of level of cognitive development" in the *Journal of Personality and Social Psychology* (1987). We thought it was a good piece of work; I still do. It did not attract much attention when it first came out; it still doesn't. What happened?

THE SEEDS FOR THE RESEARCH

As a graduate student at Arizona State University in the mid-1970s, I had been interested in attribution theory and particularly defensive attributions of responsibility. I was fascinated by the logic of the attribution process that Harold Kelley (e.g., 1973) had described in his writings about the covariation principle. The correspondence between how attribution theory said we make judgments of causality and the statistical procedures of the analysis of variance made Kelley's theory a compelling way for me to think about social perception processes. Attribution research was in many ways the start of the social cognition movement, and it offered a remarkable way to investigate how people come to understand how and why events in their world unfold as they do. As an added benefit for a new researcher like me, it was easy research to do—all you needed was paper, pencil, and a nice little scenario within which to manipulate your IVs to study the attribution processes. Life was good.

For my dissertation, I looked at cognitive consequences of accidental events: When serious accidents occur, do people become more cognitively complex as they try to understand what has transpired, or do they become more cognitively simple as they try to regain a sense of control over their circumstances? To make a sad story short, the data from my dissertation studies were not clear, and no firm conclusions could be drawn. Even hedging your bets by having competing hypotheses does not guarantee that everything will work out. But something happened in the dissertation defense that set the stage for our future research. As the committee and I engaged in the typical dissertation committee–student conversation, Bob Cialdini asked a simple question out of the blue. He asked whether causal attributions were related to subsequent behaviors. A simple question for which I had no good answer.

I wanted to say, "Well of course they do," but I could not think of any research that actually had shown that to be the case. I think everyone assumed that attributions served as guides for behavior. Fritz Heider had suggested attribution–behavior links in his "naive analysis of action" chapter. I suspect that I babbled something consistent with Heider's suggestion, but I do not know that I had much more of an answer than that. They granted me my degree anyway, and I went off to the University of Arkansas to start my career.

RESEARCH IDEAS BEGIN TO TAKE ROOT

When I started working with graduate students of my own and considered what research we should pursue, Bob's words came back to me. While I was pretty sure that attributions somehow mediated behavior (although we didn't use the term "mediate" much back then), similar assumptions about the relations between other internal, cognitive processes and overt behavior had been found to be questionable. Attitudes correlated only modestly with behavior (typical r's of 0.30–0.40); correlations between personality and behavior were of similar strength. Given that record, was there any good reason why an attribution–behavior relationship should be expected to obtain? David Johnson and I started thinking about how we might go about answering this question. In fact, in our initial attempts looking at attributions for success and failure and prescriptions for how to improve another's future performance, we found no evidence for the predicted relationship. However, being excited about null effects is not really a good way to make a point or establish a strong research program.

A few years later I was fortunate enough to have a couple of new graduate students (Lydia Walker and Judi Allen) work with me, and we decided to return to the question of attribution–behavior relations. We began to think that we might be missing some additional factor that moderated attribution–behavior relations, such that sometimes the relationship would be there and other times it would not. While there are a number of attributional phenomena in which motivational factors lead to systematic deviation from the predictions derived from attribution theory (e.g., self-serving biases, defensive attributions), we thought that there might be a cognitive reason for the failure to find attribution–behavior relations in our prior work: perhaps not all adults possess the cognitive skills necessary to make correct attributions. Some of my work had shown rather low levels of cognitive complexity among the undergraduate students who had been in our initial attribution–behavior research, and the results of a study that Dave Johnson had done suggested that not all college students had advanced to Piaget's formal-operations level of cognitive development. (I must admit that the quality of students at the University of Arkansas *at that time* might not have been the best, but they are much, much better now!) With these data-based hints as our starting point, we argued that individuals operating at Piaget's concrete-operations stage might lack the cognitive ability to integrate information and therefore to discern the correlative relations necessary to make valid causal attributions consistent with Kelley's ANOVA model.

Following this line of reasoning, Lydia Walker first took a look at whether level of cognitive development imposed a boundary condition on the application of attribution theory. Lydia found that only individuals at the formal-operations level of cognitive development were able to apply the covariation principle and to integrate relatively complex information into veridical and coherent perceptions of the roles played by possible causal factors. Concrete-operations level individuals, on the other hand, showed a marked tendency to make relatively personal causal attributions, regardless of the information provided; these subjects (we called them "subjects" back then) made attributions that were consistent with what Lee Ross labeled the fundamental attributional error. If people really transitioned into the formal-operations stage in their early teens as Piaget suggested, this might not be a big deal. However, there was evidence that a significant percentage of the adult population (perhaps as much as 50%, according to some researchers) fail to reach the formal-operations level, with the obvious implication being that as much as 50% of the adult population do not and cannot make causal attributions in the manner prescribed by Kelley and other attribution theorists.

In her thesis, Judi Allen then addressed the original question of attribution–behavior relations more directly, looking at how an attributor's level of cognitive development might affect not only the nature of the attribution made but also the manner in which those attributions are used as guides for future actions (again, in this case, improving a learner's performance on a problem-solving task). Heider had suggested that attributions allow individuals to influence distal parts of their environment. Kelley noted that causal attributions do not leave observers lost in thought, but rather the attributions guide future behavior. Ned Jones said that the particular cause that an observer identifies has important consequences for subsequent feelings and behavior. For those at the formal-operations level of cognitive development, Judi's results showed support for the claims of these theorists. Formal-operations individuals consistently prescribed a course of action to improve the learner's performance that was directly related to the causal attributions made to explain the learner's initial failure. For those at the concrete-operations level however, no reliable attribution–behavior relations were found. This lack of relationship was obtained whether the attribution used was the cause implied by the information provided to the subjects or the cause that the subject had actually chosen (right or wrong)—the subjects did not even use their own attributions as guides!

THE RESEARCH FLOWERS . . . AND THEN WITHERS ON THE VINE

We decided to combine the findings from these two studies for a submission to the *Journal of Personality and Social Psychology*. We were going to make a splash by showing the limitation of what was arguably the major social psychology theory of the day. After the inevitable revise and resubmit requests from the editor, we got the letter (a real U.S. mail letter!) accepting our paper for publication. It was published in June 1987. We waited for the accolades and citations to come rolling in. We continue to wait.

So why did our paper not have the impact that we thought or hoped that it would have? I will admit that some self-serving attributions that were none too charitable to my colleagues flashed through my mind as I considered this question. But I think there are probably at least two more valid reasons why our paper received so little attention. First, scientific contributions that show limitations and boundary conditions of theories are much less exciting than contributions that break new ground and stimulate new research ideas. Demonstrations of the generality of theories (or lack thereof) are just not that sexy; by telling readers the conditions under which a favorite theory did and did not work, we were essentially backfilling the field. When we were doing our work, attribution theory research was already a mature field, and therefore our work was not going to serve as a catalyst for new research ideas. The mother lode that Heider, Jones, and Kelley had discovered and others had successfully mined had pretty much been played out; the Zeitgeist for traditional attribution theory had passed. There might still be work to be done to clean up loose ends (as our work showed), but the time for a big splash in attribution research was gone by the time that our paper appeared in print. However, at the risk of sounding somewhat naïve or overly romantic (I do not think I am either), it should always be remembered that we are researchers in order to advance our science, not to advance our own careers. If advancing science and advancing career coincide (as they often do), that is great. But we should never forget that doing good science should always be the ultimate goal.

Second, your first word will be your last word if it is your only word. The truth is that the four of us all got involved in other professional pursuits after we had completed work on this paper, so we did not continue to pursue this line of research. After a brief stop for a temporary position at Colgate, Judi joined the faculty at Drake University and got involved in undergraduate teaching and eventually university administration. She and I published a follow-up study after this paper came out that showed high anxious/formal-operations individuals are much like concrete-operations individuals in their thinking, but that article was our last hurrah. Lydia had been in the clinical psychology program and went on to become a nationally recognized expert on domestic violence against women and children. Dave Johnson became involved with administration at his school as soon as he took his first job and then turned his attention and considerable talents to the study of teaching issues, eventually becoming the president of APA's Division 2: Society for the Teaching of Psychology. As we were working on the preparation of this manuscript, I unexpectedly became department chair, and I had already begun to shift my research attention to prosocial behavior and social dilemmas. The moral of this part of the story is that no one will be more interested in promoting the implications and extension of your work than you, and career decisions (some consciously made and others thrust upon you) inevitably mean making choices about what to pursue and what to forgo. Attribution theory and attribution–behavior relations were left behind by all four of us, but none of us was left behind. We had more to contribute to the field than just this one paper—and that might be the most important message to take away for anyone who is disappointed or discouraged that one article did not make a bigger splash.

REFERENCES

Allen, J. L., Walker, L. D., Schroeder, D. A., & Johnson, D. E. (1987). Attributions and attribution–behavior relations: The effect of level of cognitive development. *Journal of Personality and Social Psychology, 52,* 1099–1109.

Kelley, H. H. (1973). The process of causal attributions. *American Psychologist, 28,* 107–128.

PART V

Application: Making Science Useful

MARK P. ZANNA, University of Waterloo

"Risky Business": On the Adventures of Simultaneously Manipulating Sexual Arousal and Intoxication

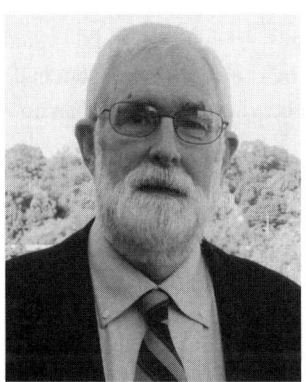

In the 1990s I became interested in applying Claude Steele's "alcohol myopia" theory (the notion that intoxication reduces cognitive capacity so that individuals are influenced primarily by cues that are momentarily salient) to solve the puzzles of (1) why men who claim to always use condoms do not always do so when intoxicated, and (2) why men who claim they would never engage in date rape might actually do so when intoxicated. In our "safe sex" research we employed a video of "boy meets girl, they go out on a date, and afterwards retire to the girl's apartment." Although it is crystal clear in the video that consensual sex is in the offing, neither has a condom. The question we asked our male participants was, in essence, if you were in this situation, would you have unprotected sex? As predicted, our participants (selected because they claimed to always use condoms) were more likely to say they'd have sex, and were more likely to indicate that "impelling" cues (such as "she's pretty") were more situationally salient than "restraining" cues (such as "she might have an STD") when they were intoxicated than when they were sober. Interestingly, in a follow-up, correlational study (MacDonald et al., 2000) we also discovered that our intoxicated participants indicated they'd have unsafe sex, but only when they also reported being sexually aroused. Thus, the important "impelling" cue in this situation turned out to be an internal one! But, of course, because we hadn't manipulated sexual arousal (but merely assessed it), we were not in a strong position to make a causal statement concerning the interaction between sexual arousal and intoxication on decision making in this (or any other) context.

As good social psychologists we began (what turned out to be) a long journey to "bottle" this interaction in the lab. In our first attempt we turned to the puzzle of why men who would never dream of committing date rape (i.e., men who rejected date rape myths) might be likely to do so when sexually aroused *and* intoxicated. Our thinking here was that such men, if aroused and intoxicated, might project their sexual arousal onto a female partner—and, thus, perceive that sex would be consensual. In our date rape research we employed a video of "boy meets girl, they go out on a date, and afterwards retire to the boy's apartment." Although it is crystal clear in the video that the boy is interested in having sex, the girl—though clearly interested in the boy—repeatedly, and clearly, says "no" to sex. The question we asked our male participants was, in essence, if you were in this situation, does "no really mean no"? This experiment was a 2 (sexual arousal: high vs. low) × 2 (intoxication: intoxicated vs. sober). In the high sexual arousal condition our male participants viewed a sexually arousing video that we created (e.g., Playboy Playmates of the Year, plus Sports Illustrated swimsuit supermodels), whereas in the low sexual arousal condition our male participants viewed an episode of "The Simpsons." The results came out exactly as we predicted (sort of). When participants reported being sexually aroused and were intoxicated, they reported the female was, in fact, interested in having consensual sex (i.e., "no didn't mean no")—and indicated various verbal and nonverbal behaviors that bolstered their judgment—to a greater extent than participants in the other three conditions that didn't differ from each other.

So why did I say "sort of"? Well, although participants did report being more sexually aroused immediately after viewing the Playmates/SI models than after viewing "The Simpsons," by the time they completed viewing the critical date rape video, the opposite was true—that is, participants reported being more sexually aroused in "The Simpsons" condition than in the Playmate/SI condition—apparently (at least, this is my best guess) because our procedure created a contrast effect! Although I was quite willing to talk about this experiment in at least four colloquia in the mid-1990s (at the University of Amsterdam, the University of Minnesota, the University of California at Santa Cruz, and Princeton University), I could never bring myself to write up a manuscript in which I would have had to include the following sentence: "Participants in the high sexual arousal condition viewed an episode of `The Simpsons,' whereas participants in the low sexual arousal condition viewed a specially edited tape of Playboy Playmates of the Year and Sports Illustrated swimsuit supermodels." Put simply, I'd decided to avoid voluntarily making myself a laughingstock—at least, in print!

But given that our hunch—that date rape might, in part, be a consequence of predictable misperceptions when men were aroused and drunk—was supported (given our twisted rationale), we decided to try again (and again) to independently manipulate sexual arousal and alcohol intoxication in the lab. First, nobody (i.e., all the female students working with me on this project) would condone my suggestion that we have an attractive female experimenter apply electrode paste (in various "sensitive" places) while our participants viewed the critical date rape video. (By the way, this suggestion was "deep-sixed" so fast I didn't even have time to figure out a cover story for why the female experimenter was applying electrode paste in the first place.) Next, we produced a version of the date rape video in which photos of Playboy Playmates were subliminally embedded each time there was a change in camera angle. Pilot-testing revealed that this manipulation (under sober conditions) made a significant difference. Unfortunately, however, male participants who viewed the standard date rape tape reported being *more* sexually aroused than male participants who viewed the tape with the embedded subliminal images of Playmates! Go figure. Well, I had absolutely no idea what to make of these results, but, needless to say, I was smart enough not to pursue them.

Although we did try other manipulations (such as leaving magazine ads with attractive models—which participants had rated in the context of a supposed different study—around when participants viewed the critical date rape video—and even spraying a mask which our participants wore with synthetic pheromones), none worked. And, when I resurrected the "electrode paste" idea (out of frustration), my suggestion was, once again, rejected "out of hand." So, for a time we put the goal of independently manipulating sexual arousal and intoxication in the lab on the back, back burner.

Instead, about a decade after our original "safe sex" research we attempted to create and test an intervention that would result in both males and females being more likely to use condoms, especially when they had been drinking, in a field experiment. Put simply, we added a cue (in the form of a friendship bracelet) designed to remind participants that they should act on their sober intentions to use condoms to a standard "safe sex" intervention. To our amazement our intervention worked, and did so to a greater extent when our participants reported they had been drinking (Dal Cin et al., 2006).

Our success with this study motivated us to try one more time to "bottle" the interaction between sexual arousal and intoxication in the lab. And fortunately Tara MacDonald finally figured out a way to do so (Ebel-Lam et al., 2009). Employing a cover story that we were interested in studying the effects of alcohol and cognitive interference on decision making, participants were told they would be reading three segments of a magazine article and viewing three scenes of a video intermittently. Those assigned to our high arousal condition read a sexually explicit story adapted from an adult magazine that described three sexual encounters between a male and female. Told from the perspective of the male character, features of the female character's body, as well as various physical encounters (e.g., kissing, touching, oral sex, and sexual intercourse), were described in explicit detail. Participants read a segment of the story, accompanied by a photograph of an attractive lingerie model, before viewing each of the three scenes of the "safe sex" video. Those assigned to the low arousal condition read three segments of an interesting story about John Glenn's return to space at age 77, accompanied by photographs of the astronaut.

Thankfully, the results were virtually identical to the results of our earlier correlational study: Compared to the other three conditions (which did not differ), our male participants who were randomly assigned to the sexual arousal condition were more likely to say they'd have unsafe sex, but only when they were intoxicated. Thus, we finally "bottled" the causal interactive effect of sexual arousal and intoxication in the lab! Needless to say, we are thankful to our Offices of Research Ethics (which allowed us to do these experiments/studies in the first place) and to all the students (RAs and actors) who worked on these studies, especially all the studies that failed!

Although persistence finally paid off, why might I expect that our final study is likely to be underappreciated? Well, put simply, because (unless someone reads this essay) no one is likely to appreciate just how hard it was to "bottle" this phenomenon. On the other hand, now that we know how to independently manipulate arousal and intoxication, it may be time to return to the lab to test our notion that men who reject date rate myths may nevertheless be inclined to commit date rape when aroused and drunk. However, given the fact that I've retired from the "alcohol business," I'll have to leave this "risky business" to more enterprising souls.

Finally, perhaps the real "take-home" message from this essay is to persist. If you have an interesting idea that turns out to be difficult to test (or to "bottle"), don't give up too early—especially if you're learning something about the phenomenon and/or the craft of experimental social psychology (e.g., how to create consequential psychological states) along the way!

REFERENCES

Dal Cin, S., MacDonald, T. K., Fong, G. T., Zanna, M. P., & Elton-Marshall, T. E. (2006). Remembering the message: Using a reminder cue to increase condom use following a safer sex intervention. *Health Psychology, 25*, 438–443.

Ebel-Lam, A. P., MacDonald, T. K., Zanna, M. P., & Fong, G. T. (2009). An experimental investigation of the interactive effects of alcohol and sexual arousal on intentions to have unprotected sex. *Basic and Applied Social Psychology, 31*, 226–233.

MacDonald, T. K., MacDonald, G., Zanna, M. P., & Fong, G. T. (2000). Alcohol, sexual arousal, and intentions to use condoms in young men: Applying alcohol myopia to risky social behavior. *Health Psychology, 19*, 290–298.

CAROL S. DWECK, Stanford University

Buried Treasures: Depression, Murder, Praise, and Intelligence

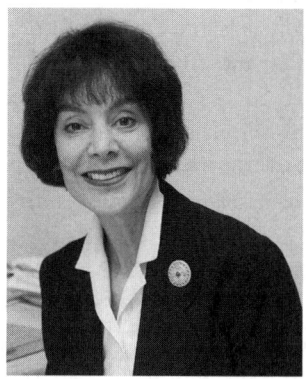

I have always believed that the editorial process is a fair one. It's an arduous one, but the outcomes over the long haul seem reasonable. I have also believed that my most important work would receive the most attention, and this too has generally been the case. However, this is the story of when things go awry.

In our work on implicit theories, we have identified the consequences of believing that people have fixed traits versus malleable qualities. We have found that thinking of one's own qualities (such as intelligence) as fixed, as opposed to malleable, leads to less challenge seeking, less persistence, more defensiveness, and lower achievement over time. We have found that thinking of *others'* traits as fixed leads to more rapid labeling and stereotyping, less openness to new information, and more punitive reactions to transgressions. And we have systematically explored the ramifications of these processes for important aspects of well-being and important arenas of human endeavor.

Yet despite the warm reception we have enjoyed over the long haul, the process doesn't always have the expected or desired result. The following are cases where the field of psychology, or the world beyond, did not embrace our work in the way we had hoped.

THE CURSE OF DEPRESSION

In one of my favorite papers, we looked at the relation between people's implicit theories and depression. If implicit theories could be linked to depression, it might have implications for how depression could be treated or prevented. In several studies, we found that the more qualities people saw as fixed, the more readily they recalled negative events, the more helpless were their reactions to negative events, and the greater was their reported depression. Although this research did not establish a causal connection between implicit theories and depression, it was a nice start. Reviewers—all of them—loved the paper and hailed it as a contribution. Editors, however, withheld their blessing.

We approached the question again a few years later. This time we looked at the impact of the chronic goals that are typically associated with implicit theories—the goal of attempting to validate oneself, which is typically linked to the fixed theory, versus the goal of growth, which is typically linked to the malleable theory. Using a killer combination of daily diary and experimental methods, we not only found that goals predicted depression but also showed that negative affect had a completely different effect within each goal. With strong validation goals, the more depressed affect college students reported, the less they engaged in problem solving when things went wrong. This is how we typically think of depression. However, with strong growth goals, the more depressed affect they reported, the *more* they engaged in problem solving in the face of negative events. Depressed affect seemed to energize them!

And then we showed the same thing experimentally by manipulating people's goals, measuring their depressed affect after a failure, and showing increased or decreased problem solving. Again within the validation goal, a higher level of negative affect predicted poorer problem solving, compared to the growth goal, in which a higher level of negative affect predicted better problem solving. Who could resist this paper? Not the reviewers—once again they loved it. And once again, the editors failed to heed their advice.

We found something valuable, but it did not follow in the footsteps of my other contributions. I hope that the negative affect that the process engendered in us, like the negative affect in our growth-oriented participants, will fuel further problem solving. But enough about depression—let's move on to murder and guilt!

JUDGING A DEFENDANT'S GUILT OR INNOCENCE

I have told you how people with a fixed theory label and judge people very rapidly, often on the basis of very sparse information. They may see even superficial aspects of a person's appearance or behavior as deeply meaningful and as informative about basic underlying traits. People with a malleable theory of human qualities, in contrast, do not believe in fixed traits and, although they take notice of appearance and behavior, they do not invest it with magical diagnostic significance.

In two studies, Ben Gervey, C. Y. Chiu, Ying-yi Hong, and I (1999) showed that people's theories could tell us when (and why) they would convict a man of murder. We gave people an abbreviated transcript of a murder trial. In one condition, the defendant, on the day of the murder, was wearing or doing something respectable—he was wearing a business suit (Study 1) or was seen leaving the public library (Study 2). In the other condition he was wearing or doing something less respectable—he was wearing a leather jacket full of chains (Study 1) or was seen leaving an adult bookstore (Study 2). We found that, first, people with the fixed view consistently rated the less respectable guy as less moral and trustworthy. They also convicted him of the murder at a much higher rate than they convicted the respectable guy. Moreover, they were far more likely to ignore potentially exonerating evidence. That is, their belief in the telltale nature of his appearance and behavior completely overrode the actual evidence.

People with the malleable view, however, did not place much stock in the information about the defendant's appearance or prior behavior. Their ratings of the defendant's morality were not affected by his garb or his reading matter. However, their verdicts *were* affected by the evidence itself. In other words, those with the malleable theory appeared to be constructing a coherent narrative of what happened the day of the murder and not a story about the underlying fixed goodness or evil of the defendant.

These findings have interesting implications for the judicial process. They suggest that different kinds of evidence will be compelling to jurors with different implicit theories. If the jury has a preponderance of people with a fixed view, it would be particularly important to address issues of character. However, if the jury has a preponderance of people with a malleable view, it would be particularly important to build a coherent and persuasive narrative for them. The findings also suggest that juries might sometimes be deadlocked not because they disagree about the evidence presented but because they are using different criteria to weigh that evidence and to judge the case.

Surely these findings would cause a stir, but not even a ripple has been detected as yet. Maybe this work was not done in the tradition of the typical jury study. Maybe we wrote it up more as a finding about implicit theories than about jury decision making. Maybe it was published before the days in which the world took heed of psychologists' noteworthy findings. But there's still hope. Maybe Bob Arkin will edit a volume of all the neglected studies lamented in this book and give them another chance!

MAKING A DIFFERENCE

Sometimes we do work that is relevant to people's lives and that, if put into practice, could do some good. I have been extremely fortunate that much of my work has reached the public and has made an impact. But I have been amazed at what a difficult and haphazard process this is. In 1998, Claudia Mueller and I published a paper on the perils of praise. In six studies, we showed that praise for intelligence undermined children's motivation and performance, whereas praise for process (e.g., effort) could enhance them. It punched a big hole in the argument of the self-esteem movement that the more praise and the more global the praise, the better it would be for the child. Our findings received a great deal of recognition and were covered by many major newspapers, magazines, and news programs around the country and beyond. And that was that. After a brief, intense period of attention, it faded from public consciousness and parents were still praising their children's intelligence and talent to the skies even as the spark went out of their children's eyes. It was not until 9 years later, when a cover story in a big-time magazine sounded the alarm and jolted parents into paying attention, that our findings began to be more widely influential. It was then that parents started talking among themselves and began to consider the possibility that praising children's intelligence was not the defining feature of a good parent. It was then that they began to form support groups to help each other break the habit.

The same thing happened with our work on implicit theories of intelligence. We had been doing studies for years on the drawbacks of a fixed theory and the benefits of a malleable theory, and it had been written about in the press. Yet only when NPR's *Morning Edition* and *Good Morning America* covered the work in the same week did people at large sit up, take notice, and begin to apply the lessons of this work in the real world.

I have tried to do my part in this endeavor. I have written a book, *Mindset*, for the public. I have written extensively for education, business, and sports publications. I have given numerous talks to numerous real-world groups. But it is a difficult process. Why is that? First, as I suggest above, it is hard to get a big enough platform to reach a large number of people. But perhaps even more important, I have come to realize that much of the public does not understand why research is special. They do not quite grasp why someone with good evidence should be heeded more than a charismatic guru who simply has conviction.

I believe we have a big task before us: to educate the public that putting *tested* ideas into practice is a good idea—and that any idea that is put into practice on a large scale should be evaluated. Right now we have huge innovations occurring in education and business, but they are often haphazard or fad-driven. Someone should be evaluating the existing research evidence before these giant steps are taken or, at the very least, taking these steps in a way that can tell us which initiatives worked and which did not. Or which worked for certain people, groups, or organizations and which worked for others.

CONCLUSION

This book is about hardships. It is about papers unpublished, papers unappreciated by the field, and work that does not reach the public. However, the message ought not be a discouraging one. We should instead take a malleable view. It is an imperfect world, but perhaps, with effort, we can reshape it. This book takes a nice step in that direction.

REFERENCES

Gervey, B., Chiu, C., Hong, Y., & Dweck, C. S. (1999). Differential use of person information in decision-making about guilt vs. innocence: The role of implicit theories. *Personality and Social Psychology Bulletin, 25*, 17–27.

Mueller, C. M., & Dweck, C. S. (1998). Intelligence praise can undermine motivation and performance. *Journal of Personality and Social Psychology, 75*, 33–52.

ALICE H. EAGLY, Northwestern University

A Mis-citation Classic

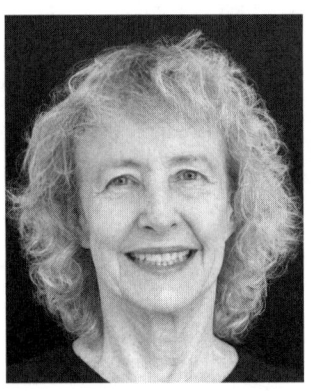

I published an article in 1995 in *Psychological Bulletin* titled "Gender and the effectiveness of leaders: A meta-analysis," co-authored with Steven J. Karau and Mona G. Makhijani. The article addressed the very important question of whether female and male leaders differ in effectiveness. This article has been moderately successful, so far cited 177 times according to Web of Science. Although fame and fortune have not followed from this publication, it has achieved good dissemination.

So what is the problem? The issue is that the findings of our review are often cited as making a point that is contrary to the central theme of the article. This outcome is disheartening, given all of the work that went into producing an excellent quantitative synthesis. Meta-analyses are meant to keep us from, often unknowingly, selectively citing findings that match our preconceptions. The meta-analyst is supposed to be an honest broker who mediates between the research literature and researchers and activists whose theoretical and ideological agendas lead them to prefer certain types of findings. Therefore, the meta-analyst locates all of the studies that tested a given hypothesis, preferably including dissertations, conference papers, and gray literature. There are sometimes many such relatively hidden studies that have not been published in normal channels, often due to weak or nonsignificant findings. The "truth" of an effect emerges from examining and evaluating all appropriately designed and implemented tests, not just those whose significant and interesting findings yielded publication in good journals. These goals of meta-analysis are admirable but do not allow for readers' ability to massage the findings of these reviews to conform to their preconceptions.

To understand how meta-analyses allow such misunderstandings, consider the details of our 1995 *Psychological Bulletin* article. This meta-analysis presented the results of 96 studies that had compared the effectiveness of male and female leaders, predominantly managers in organizational settings but also including some leaders in laboratory studies. Most of the dependent measures consisted of subjective performance appraisals, although some objective outcome measures were also present in these studies.

What were our main findings? We found heterogeneous effects ranging from those in which men were more effective than women to those in which women were more effective than men. Our task then became sorting out these findings with moderator variables that accounted for this variability in outcomes. We were successful in this task, aided mainly by a straightforward role incongruity hypothesis postulating that leaders fare better if their leader role is congruent with their gender—that is, male leaders are rated more favorably in more culturally masculine leader roles and female leaders in less masculine leader roles. We evaluated these cultural aspects of the leader roles by having student raters judge the roles in the reviewed studies from a brief description of each role. Consistent with our role incongruity hypothesis, these ratings tracked the findings in the expected manner. A related analysis found that men were especially more effective than women in military settings, and women slightly more effective than men in governmental, social service, and educational settings. The results of this categorization by setting also made sense according to our role incongruity hypothesis, which emphasizes the perceived fit between group stereotypes and the requirements of social roles.

Our meta-analysis also produced an overall mean sex comparison on effectiveness, and therein lies our problem. This mean effect size averaged over all of the comparisons between male and female leaders is arbitrary because its value depended on the types of studies that we were able to find and include in the meta-analysis. We did not have a sample of studies representative of all settings in which people occupy leadership roles. If the sample had included many military studies, this mean value would have been pushed to favor men; if the sample had included many governmental, social service, and educational studies, the mean would have been pushed to favor women. Given the particular studies we found, the mean effect size was near zero, with a d effect size of -0.02.

Given these findings, one rendition of our results is merely that men and women are equally effective as leaders. However, equal effectiveness was not present in most of the studies. Our null aggregate outcome meant that the studies with the more masculine leader roles happened to have almost perfectly balanced the studies with the less masculine leadership roles, to produce the near-zero mean. The important conclusion of the project is that context is all-important and that both women and men have advantage in roles that are culturally more congenial to their own sex.

Many writers have entirely missed our main point. For example, Powell and Ansic (1997, p. 607) wrote that "Males and females are found to be ... equally effective in leadership roles" (Eagly et al., 1995). Many such authors followed such a statement with a simple gender similarity argument that women are just as good leaders as men, presumably in all settings, and therefore any lack of women in leader roles is due to discrimination. Discrimination is surely often present in relation to women as leaders. However, the stance that women and men are always equally effective is far too simple because people do face special challenges to their effectiveness in organizational settings defined by the other sex. These challenges are especially great for women in extremely masculine settings such as the military, as suggested by our findings. Unfortunately, many researchers who cited our meta-analysis have completely ignored this generalization about role incongruity, which took up most of the article, in the predictions, the description of the findings, and the theoretical analysis.

It is true that quite a few other citations of the meta-analysis have stated the findings correctly. For example, Gutek (2001, p. 382) wrote that "men are particularly effective in leadership roles stereotyped as congenial to men, and women are especially effective in roles stereotyped as congenial to women." Nonetheless, the many citations claiming that we have proven that men and women do not differ in effectiveness show that it can be difficult to convey complex findings.

Were these misunderstandings actually our fault? To some extent, we are guilty because the second sentence of our abstract indicated that "Aggregated over the organizational and laboratory experimental studies in the sample, male and female leaders were equally effective" (Eagly et al., 1995, p. 125). Yet, the next word in the abstract was "However," and the remainder of the abstract detailed the role incongruity findings. Also, the beginning of the Results section and first paragraph of the Discussion section presented the overall "no difference" mean finding. However, the remainder of the Results and Discussion sections provided a detailed consideration of the moderation that we obtained. We also explicitly warned readers that a generalization about male–female equivalence is not valid in many organizational settings, as demonstrated by the strong context effects we obtained.

In retrospect, how might we have presented our findings? One possibility is to have given very little emphasis to the overall mean of the effects, perhaps presenting it only after presenting the strong moderators. However, the convention in meta-analytic articles is to first give information about the mean and distribution of the effects, and only then to follow it with the moderators. Presenting moderators first and then the overall mean no doubt would have been confusing to readers. More realistically, we might have issued stronger warnings about the arbitrariness of the near-zero overall mean and stronger directives that the demonstration of role incongruity is the important aspect of the data. This warning should have been present in the abstract as well as the body of the article, especially at the beginning of the Discussion section.

To the extent that I have learned something from our mis-citation classic, that lesson is to be wary about who might cite an article in the future and therefore to think about what his or her agenda might be. I should have realized that the "no difference" overall mean finding would be very attractive to many readers because of its seemingly desirable, if simple-minded, implications for gender equality. It was thus not only the complexity of our findings that favored mis-citation but the particular mindset of many of our readers, who are committed to furthering gender equality. However, to make genuine progress toward gender equality, both researchers and activists must confront the challenges of role-incongruent settings, not paper over them.

REFERENCES

Eagly, A. H., Karau, S. J., & Makhijani, M. G. (1995). Gender and the effectiveness of leaders: A meta-analysis. *Psychological Bulletin, 117*, 125–145.

Gutek, B. (2001). Women and paid work. (2001). *Psychology of Women Quarterly, 25*, 379–393.

Powell, M., & Ansic, D. (1997). Gender differences in risk behaviour in financial decision-making: An experimental analysis. *Journal of Economic Psychology, 18*, 605–628.

PETER SALOVEY, Yale University

Emotional Intelligence

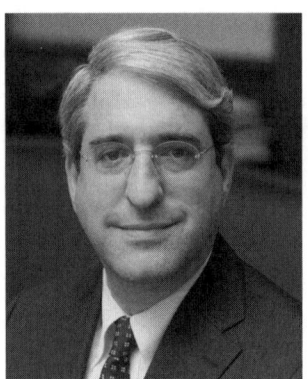

In recent years, the phrase *emotional intelligence* appeared in the comic strips "Dil-bert" and "Zippy the Pinhead" as well as higher-brow humorous fare by Roz Chast in the *New Yorker*. And in the mid-1990s, *emotional intelligence* was named the most useful new word or phrase by the American Dialect Society. There are now tens of thousands of references to emotional intelligence in journals and websites devoted to psychology, education, and organizational behavior.

But it wasn't always this way. When John D. (Jack) Mayer and I wrote our first manuscript on emotional intelligence, we were concerned that we would not be able to get it published. The initial reaction to the idea was decidedly hostile.

Jack Mayer and I met and became friends over our shared interest in the effects of mood and emotion on cognitive processes. Jack had been a postdoctoral fellow with Gordon Bower at Stanford University and collaborated with him on classic work concerning mood state-dependent memory. Some years earlier, I had been an under-graduate at Stanford, and in David Rosenhan's laboratory had conducted a couple of studies testing the interaction of mood and attentional focus on helping behavior. In the summer of 1987, Jack (then on the faculty of the State University of New York at Purchase) came up to New Haven to help me paint the interior of a house that my wife and I had just purchased. And while painting, we talked a bit about research in person-ality-social psychology.

Jack had cut his teeth in the area of human intelligence, and I identified as an emo-tions researcher. Applying a second coat of eggshell finish to the living room wall, Jack lamented that theories of intelligence hadn't really ever focused in a systematic way on a place for emotion—Howard Gardner's *intrapersonal intelligence* notwithstanding—and I complained that investigators of human emotion seemed not to have much interest in individual differences in the ways people approached their own and others' emotions or the influence of emotion on thinking. And so the idea of *emotional intel-ligence* was born; perhaps Jack was the first actually to utter the phrase.

In any case, we began to talk through the idea of an emotional intelligence—What would be the underlying capacities? How would it be adaptive?—and we considered whether we should try to put all this on paper. Sometime later, an opportunity to attend a small social psychology conference at Bibb Latane's Nags Head, North Car-olina, beach house provided the chance to sketch out a manuscript describing emo-tional intelligence. This paper began with what we thought was a clever opening sentence: "Is 'emotional intelligence' a contradiction in terms?" We then went on to present a framework describing "a set of skills hypothesized to contribute to the accurate appraisal and expression of emotion in oneself and others, the effective regulation of emotion in self and others, and the use of feelings to motivate, plan, and achieve in one's life" (Salovey & Mayer, 1990, p. 185). And we offered up a concep-tual definition of emotional intelligence as an individual's capacity to reason about emotions and to process emotional information in order to enhance reasoning.

The manuscript, which we titled simply *Emotional Intelligence*, began to take shape in 1988 and, after eliciting comments on it from colleagues and friends, we submitted it to well-read psychology journals that publish broad conceptual articles intended for wide audiences. I cannot bring myself to describe the unenthusiastic responses we received, and I won't try to quote them verbatim. Essentially, review-ers either obsessed that nothing we were describing sounded at all like "an intelli-gence" or that the field of emotions research would not be advantaged by focusing on individual differences, let alone co-mingling its ideas with the problematic con-cept of "intelligence." Jack and I were disappointed by this outcome (and took no pleasure in how promptly we received the unambiguous feedback).

Not knowing what to do with the manuscript, and wondering if the problem was that we had stumbled on a truly stupid idea, we asked my senior colleague at Yale, Jerome L. Singer, to read the paper and provide feedback. (As it happens, when Jack was a boy, his family lived in the same neighborhood of Ardsley, New York, as the Singers, and the two families knew each other; the children played together.) Jerry read the paper, gave us very thoughtful feedback and told us that he would like us to submit it to a journal he edited, *Imagination, Cognition, and Personality*. And so we revised the manuscript and submitted it to him. Some months later, after sending it out for review and a bit more revising on our part, the paper was accepted and appeared in print in 1990 (Salovey & Mayer, 1990). Although the phrase *emotional intelligence* could be found here and there prior to the publication of our 1990 article—in a book on literary criticism, in a German piece on motherhood, in a dissertation—the paper published in *Imagination, Cognition, and Personality* is considered the first scientific definition and systematic use of the phrase.

It's been 20 years since the publication of that paper, and Jack and I are proud that it is the most cited article ever published in *Imagination, Cognition, and Personality*. And, despite its appearance in a rather small journal not even included in the Web of Science database, it is far and away the most cited paper either Jack or I have written: According to Google Scholar this morning, it has been cited nearly 3,000 times.

In the first few years after *Emotional Intelligence* appeared, however, it was hardly cited at all. It took a very unusual event to put our 1990 paper on the map. The journalist and psychologist Daniel Goleman published a book in the fall of 1995 called *Emotional Intelligence,* which went on to sell millions of copies worldwide, rising to #2 on the *New York Times* bestseller list and remaining on the list for more than a year. The book received enormous media attention following its publication, with cover stories in *Time Magazine, USA Today Magazine,* and publications all over the world. I had presented our emotional intelligence framework at a conference organized by Goleman a couple of years earlier, and he told me that he liked the idea and was considering it for the title of a book he was writing. When the book appeared, he graciously cited our work and indicated in the acknowledgments that he had first learned of the term when I gave him the 1990 article.

Goleman's book—still the most readable discussion of emotional intelligence written for a general audience—brought considerable attention to research on emotional intelligence (indeed, on human emotion more generally), especially as the media began to view emotional intelligence as a kind of magic bullet that would solve problems in schools, workplaces, and families. Of course, at the time his book appeared, no one had yet proposed a way to measure emotional intelligence. But this did not stop the media, and even some people who should have known better, from suggesting it is more important than IQ and accounts for huge percentages of the variance in significant outcomes; the *Time Magazine* cover story declared "emotional intelligence may be the best predictor of success in life, redefining what it means to be smart."

For Jack and me, we realized that we needed to take seriously an idea that we had really proposed as a kind of thought experiment. We hadn't originally intended on describing emotional intelligence in a more precise way, but soon updated our framework to make it more operational (Mayer & Salovey, 1997). And, after criticizing the disappointing ways in which some were proposing to measure emotional intelligence (e.g., with self-report inventories containing items like, "I am usually aware of others' feelings"), we got to work with our colleague David Caruso developing an ability-based measure of emotional intelligence that would hold up psychometrically (Mayer, Salovey, Caruso, & Sitarenios, 2003).

There is now a growing literature on emotional intelligence testing its predictive validity, and such studies are yielding promising findings (Mayer, Salovey, & Caruso,

2008). The idea remains of considerable interest to schools desiring to add social and emotional learning (SEL) to the curriculum as well as to organizations hoping to develop the skills of their managers. Nonetheless, the idea remains unloved in certain circles. For instance, some leaders in the organizational behavior field declared it "preposterously all encompassing," an "invalid concept," and "outside the typical scientific domain;" earlier reaction to it in personality-social psychology used words like "elusive" and "more myth than science." We believe this reaction to the idea of emotional intelligence was partly due to confusion between what had been said about it in the scientific literature with what had been declared in media representations and books written for general audiences. More importantly, attempts to measure emotional intelligence in (self-reported) trait terms rather than as a set of abilities led to the problem that it appeared not to be well differentiated from more familiar concepts such as subjective well-being or the Big Five model of personality.

It is our belief, however, that as research continues to appear in which investigators test the validity of emotional intelligence (measured as a set of abilities) to predict important social outcomes over and above personality constructs and traditionally measured IQ, and others continue to develop methods for improving these skills among children and adults, the promise of emotional intelligence will become more obvious and the criticisms will be less dismissive and—appropriately—more focused on how best to define, assess, and improve these competences.

Are there general lessons to be learned from this story? Well, the obvious one—indeed, one of the "take-home points" of this entire book—is to stick with ideas even when they don't seem especially popular. Although the fact that no one has investigated some phenomenon does not automatically mean it is a good one to explore, it is also the case that ideas that are unpopular at one time and in one context might prove more useful later and in unintended ways. Second, once an idea receives attention in the general media—and the Internet allows ideas to "go viral" with greater facility than was the case in the early 1990s—it becomes very difficult to maintain any kind of discipline with respect to how a construct is defined, operationalized, or used. The genie is out of the bottle, I'm afraid, and stuffing it back in is futile. All one can do is to try to maintain some kind of objective distance from the hoopla and avoid compromising one's own scientific integrity in an attempt to feed the frenzy. Third, and despite what I have just said, if an unloved idea suddenly gains popularity, try to enjoy it! In the late 1990s, following the publication of Goleman's book, Jack, David, and I had the opportunity to travel the world speaking about emotional intelligence and developing interesting research collaborations. Nothing wrong with that! Finally, don't neglect the wisdom, support, and encouragement that friends and colleagues can provide during difficult moments, especially when all appears hopeless. Jack and I try not to let too much time pass without thanking Jerry Singer, whose enthusiasm for the idea of emotional intelligence and encouragement to publish our first paper in his journal in fact changed our lives. We hope it has had a similar effect on the field, but that is for others to decide.

REFERENCES

Mayer, J. D., & Salovey, P. (1997). What is emotional intelligence? In P. Salovey & D. Sluyter (Eds.), *Emotional development and emotional intelligence: Implications for educators* (pp. 3–31). New York: Basic Books.

Mayer, J. D., Salovey, P., & Caruso, D. R. (2008). Emotional intelligence: New ability or eclectic traits? *American Psychologist, 63,* 503–517.

Mayer, J. D., Salovey, P., Caruso, D. R., & Sitarenios, G. (2003). Measuring emotional intelligence with the MSCEIT V2.0. *Emotion, 3,* 97–105.

Salovey, P., & Mayer, J.D. (1990). Emotional intelligence. *Imagination, Cognition, and Personality, 9,* 185–211.

TOM R. TYLER, New York University

Hidden Gems About Justice Research: The Psychology of Punitiveness

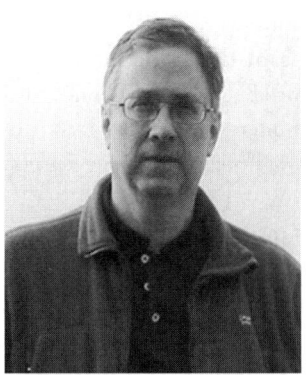

I am fortunate to have been a graduate student at UCLA and in the lab of David Sears. There are many reasons why this was an unusual opportunity, two of which are relevant to the topic of this volume. First, David has a very broad vision of social science and encourages his students to learn the theories and methodologies of all of the social sciences, not just social psychology, so it becomes natural to think about writing and publishing in a broader range of journals than are considered by many psychologists. Second, when I was a student David was in the process of developing the ideas about symbolic politics that have subsequently become widely influential in public policy. I was lucky to be present at the creation and, as a consequence, involved in many of the discussions in which these ideas were first framed. Without the encouragement and support that I received in the Sears lab as a graduate student I doubt that I would have been able to develop a career that addresses both theories in social psychology and the public policy implications of those theories.

The central idea underlying symbolic politics is that people's policy positions are not driven by their personal or group-based interests. In contrast to the widely articulated rational choice model, in other words, people do not advocate or support issues positions because those positions advance their own material interests.

For example, people with young children are not those who fight school integration, nor are those without homes the primary supporters of property tax increases. Rather, people's policy positions are a response to their political ideologies (Sears, Lau, Tyler, & Allen, 1980). Since David's concerns are political, his studies make heavy use of political ideology and party membership.

In my own work I have found this symbolic perspective to be a valuable starting point for exploring issues related to law and criminal justice. For example, in an early study on support for the death penalty (Tyler & Weber, 1982-83), Renee Weber and I found that support for punitive public policies such as the death penalty is not linked particularly strongly to whether people have been crime victims; whether they fear future crime victimization; or even whether they think crime is a major problem in their communities. Rather, support for the death penalty is primarily a consequence of the core social value of authoritarianism. And, as social psychologists have made clear ever since the foundational work of Adorno authoritarianism is a fundamental human value that people learn early in life and that persists across adulthood. These findings fit very comfortably within the conceptual framework of symbolic politics by showing that self-interest does not shape people's views about desirable public policies; rather, those policy positions develop out of fundamental social values.

Although the argument that self-interest does not matter is an important one, a demonstration that something else *does matter* has to be central to efforts at generating further interest among scholars and policy makers. To some extent focusing on values addresses this question, but, since social psychologists present an image of values as developed in childhood and generally unchanging after that, it is difficult to identify an action strategy that flows from viewing policy positions as linked to social values. The clearest strategy that follows is an extremely long-term one: for instance, focus on socializing the next generation with better values and waiting until they become adults for policies to change.

In an effort to better understand the psychology of punitiveness and to identify a more compelling strategy for social change, I further explored policy support in California in the context of the highly punitive "three-strikes law." That law, passed in 1994, mandates life in prison for those convicted of three felonies. At the time it was proposed, this ballot initiative was almost universally opposed by legal authorities, and its passage is a direct reflection of the strength of public feeling on this issue at the time. This feeling was widely framed in the public discourse in terms of the issue of fear of crime. However, I have argued that fear of crime is not the root of public punitiveness.

The prison population of California increased substantially after the three-strikes law passed, and the state incurred enormous costs associated with building, staffing and otherwise maintaining this large set of public institutions. Today the three-strikes law is being reconsidered, but for budget reasons, not due to a general revision in public sentiment about criminals. And even in the dire economic times we are now living through, such proposals face an uncertain fate. For example, proposals to make the draconian drug laws in New York State more lenient have confronted strong opposition even in the face of evidence that sustaining them will have dire consequences for other programs in this cash-strapped state. Whatever happens at this time, it is easy to imagine that when economic pressures lessen, pressure for punitiveness will re-emerge.

In the study I will discuss (Tyler & Boeckmann, 1997), Robert Boeckmann and I explored the non-instrumental reasons that people had for supporting this punitive initiative. We also looked beyond support for the initiative and considered support for punitive policies in general. Our results support a very social psychological perspective on punishment. We found two sources of support for punitiveness. First, values shape punitiveness directly, as we know from prior studies: More dogmatic and authoritarian people are more punitive.

But punitiveness is also related to judgments about the social environment: the belief that the world is dangerous and the belief that the world is not morally cohesive. In other words, punitiveness is linked to judgments concerning the nature of society. In particular, people are concerned about issues of the family and of diversity. In the case of the family, people believe that the family is declining and that parents no longer teach their children moral and social values. As a consequence, young people are dangerous and out of control. This feeling is intensified by issues of diversity. As society becomes more diverse (and California is a very diverse state) people increasingly believe that there are few shared values that unite people into one community. As a consequence, it is more difficult to appeal to shared values for purposes of shaming or rehabilitation. Without moral values or social ties to use as a basis for changing lawbreakers, there are few viable alternatives to simply warehousing offenders.

I think these findings are important because they advance our understanding of the psychology underlying punitiveness, and hence help us to understand how to approach trying to change public views. An understanding of why people support punitive policies provides a basis for developing strategies for addressing public concerns and thereby lessening the feelings that lead to support for punitive public policies.

The need to address public feelings has become increasingly important as the United States has become ever more distinctive in the world for the dramatically large proportion of its population that it has in prison. Today, the United States is a world leader in the proportion of citizens it holds in prison. In 2000, there were over 2 million Americans in jail or prison, far surpassing incarceration rates in Europe and elsewhere. Recently the Pew Center on the States made headlines by indicating that 1 in 100 are behind bars in the United States (Pew Center, 2008). Those policies have monetary costs, but they are also responsible for destroying lives and communities, in particular the minority-based inner-city communities, in which the members of almost every family and household have been or are incarcerated.

While there have been calls for reductions in punitiveness that are framed in terms of the costs of the prison system in an era of fiscal austerity, it is striking that such calls do not reflect any change in the attitudes toward criminals. Rather, they reflect the desire for a temporary change in policies until the economic picture improves. Studies of public opinion suggest that public punitiveness remains strong, so these are calls for a temporary accommodation to scarcities. To make a more fundamental and long-lasting change, we need to understand why Americans are so strongly and uniquely punitive. The study I mentioned shows that psychologists can make a useful contribution to this effort, although at this time our voice has been largely missing from these discussions. Certainly my work in this area, reflected in that study, has not inspired much such effort on the part of psychologists.

So, to summarize, this paper on the three-strikes law is the focus of my comments on underappreciated ideas because I think it has good ideas, but I acknowledge that it has had little influence upon social psychological research.

In my view one reason for this general lack of influence is the placement of this paper. Because it is based upon correlational data collected in a survey and because of the issues it addresses, this study found its home in a social science journal rather than in a social psychology venue. This is not to say that social psychology journals do not publish correlational data, but they have a more restricted focus upon issues of causality that considers only certain types of research efforts to be "good science." They also publish research that speaks to public policy concerns, but primarily in journals that are "applied" and where having work published condemns that work to second-class status. This restricted focus makes sense in terms of internal validity, but it means that many social psychological papers lack the type of external validity that would lead their findings to be more relevant to and more likely to be used by people making policy decisions. As an example, experiments show that something can be influential, but they do not indicate the range and strength of its influence in natural settings, information central to making policy tradeoffs.

My suggestion is that by having such a restricted conceptual and methodological focus, social psychology has prevented itself from weighing in on some of the major public policy issues of our day. This is especially disappointing since, from my point of view, social psychology has a lot to say about those issues, and I modestly put my paper forward as one example of such a case of neglected good ideas. Of course, I also acknowledge that I am not the only person trying to bring theoretical ideas about punishment to bear on public policy issues: Darley and Robinson are dealing with the same issues I am raising here (Robinson & Darley, 1995, 2004).

As is becoming increasingly clear, our society, and perhaps more importantly the funding agencies that our society supports, ever more frequently raise questions about why they should support "esoteric" research that does not speak to important societal concerns. Hence, social psychologists have a lot to gain by expanding their conceptual and methodological nets. Society has a lot to gain also, since I think social psychology has more sophisticated ideas in many areas of public policy than those that currently dominate our social institutions. And, of course, I would gain too, since people might then pay more attention to my favorite underappreciated study.

REFERENCES

Pew Center for the States. (2008). *One in 100: Behind Bars in America.*

Robinson, P. H., & Darley, J. (1995). *Justice, liability, and blame.* Boulder, CO: Westview.

Robinson, P. H., & Darley, J. (2004). Does criminal law deter? A behavioural science investigation. *Oxford Journal of Legal Studies, 24,* 173–205.

Sears, D. O., Lau, R. R., Tyler, T. R., & Allen, H. M., Jr. (1980). Self-interest and symbolic politics in policy attitudes and Presidential voting. *American Political Science Review, 74,* 670–684.

Tyler, T. R., & Weber, R. (1982-83). Support for the death penalty: Instrumental response to crime or symbolic attitude? *Law and Society Review, 17,* 201–224.

Tyler, T. R., & Boeckmann, R. (1997). Three strikes and you are out, but why? The psychology of public support for punishing rule breakers. *Law and Society Review, 31,* 237–265.

SAUL M. KASSIN, John Jay College of Criminal Justice
The "Messenger Effect" in Persuasion

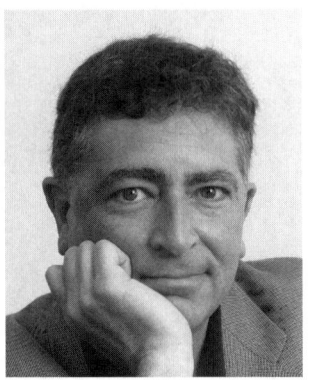

I can think of a number of reasons why any one of us would consider a piece of our own research "underappreciated": It was never accepted for publication and should have been; it was published but drew insufficient attention (perhaps because the author was obscure at the time, the topic was not hot or "in the air," or the article appeared in a second-tier journal); it was published and drew the scant attention it deserved—and our opinions are, quite simply, inflated and out of step with reality.

Mindful of the more-or-less flattering, if not derogatory, attributions that could be hurled at my hidden gem, I will take the risk and proceed anyway. My story begins in 1981. Three years out of graduate school, I was beginning to transition from basic social psychology (my graduate work at the University of Connecticut, with Skip Lowe, studying attribution theory and biases) into applications to juries, evidence, and other aspects of law (as a result of a postdoctoral fellowship with Larry Wrightsman at the University of Kansas).

The inspiration for my underappreciated gem can be traced to a phone call I received from Chicago-based attorneys representing more than 40,000 consumers in a class-action suit against General Motors. At the time, this case was referred to in the media as the "Chevymobile" engine switch case. Apparently, GM had installed inferior Chevrolet engines rather than the usual Oldsmobile "Rocket" 350 engines in various high-end models, and consumers were taking GM to trial. In preparation for their jury trial, the lawyers contacted me, and we conducted a one-day mock trial in a federal courtroom. Four lawyers presented the case for both sides, an actual judge presided over the proceedings, three witnesses testified live, the testimony of six witnesses who had been deposed was read into the record from the witness stand, and 18 jury-eligible citizens filled out questionnaires and then deliberated to a verdict in three six-person groups (for more information about this case, see Kassin [1984]).

The data obtained from the mock juries were eminently useful to the plaintiffs' attorneys. Then something odd happened. Two weeks before trial, I received a phone call from these attorneys: "We are auditioning professional actors and actresses from Actors' Equity this Saturday to play the role of missing witnesses. Are you interested?" Apparently, the plaintiffs had deposed several witnesses, including GM executives, who for one reason or another would not appear at trial. The technophobic judge in the case refused to allow videotaped testimony of any kind in his courtroom, so the plaintiffs had to resort to the conventional method of reading a transcript of the deposition into the record—the attorney reading the questions, an individual appointed by the attorney, seated in the witness stand, reading the answers (for a more detailed discussion of the procedure, see Kassin & Wrightsman [1988]).

What an opportunity for mischief this procedure presented! Knowing they could appoint anyone to read for a missing witness, the attorneys auditioned professionals and told them what kind of impression they wanted to convey of their witness. I will never forget my puzzlement at seeing attorneys pre-instruct one actress before she read the part of a GM executive to make that witness appear uncooperative (I believe but will not swear that the word "bitch" was used). She was masterful and quite nuanced in her performance. By pausing at just the right moments, crossing her legs, rolling her eyes, and sighing before delivering her scripted answers, she was able to portray the witness in dislikable terms—all the while staying faithful to the spoken word. I kept asking the lawyers, are you sure you are permitted to replace a witness with an actor seeking to create a specific positive or negative impression? The answer was yes. Sure enough, those actors and actresses who won parts took to the witness stand in a Chicago courtroom. Ultimately, the plaintiffs prevailed.

Stunned by what I had seen, I wondered if hired guns substituting for absentee witnesses could truly taint a jury's perceptions of those witnesses. The jury was carefully instructed before each deposition reading that the individual on the stand was not the witness but merely someone reading the real witness's sworn testimony. Were they influenced nevertheless by the reader's demeanor? Or, were they capable of making the correction to discount the delivery of the testimony, as opposed to its content? I combed through the vast warehouse of research on attitudes and persuasion, beginning with the post-World War II work of the Yale Group through the most recent studies representing the early work on ELM. Nothing. The research literature was silent. Sure, there was the long tradition of research on source effects in persuasion. Remarkably, however, no distinction was ever made between communicators who are the origin or *source* of the message they deliver and those who are mere *messengers* for the source. The attribution theorist in me was dumbfounded by what seemed like a gaping hole.

Is it truly possible to alter a jury's impression of an absentee witness by altering the reader's demeanor? To test this hypothesis, I conducted a mock jury experiment and published the results in *PSPB* in a paper entitled "Deposition testimony and the surrogate witness: Evidence for a 'messenger effect' in persuasion" (Kassin, 1983). Participants were presented with a civil suit that hinged largely on the testimony of a target witness. I hired a professional actor to play that role in one of two ways on videotape. In a positive demeanor condition, he was attentive, polite, unhesitant, and unwavering in his style. In a negative demeanor condition, the same actor reading from the same transcript was impolite, often appearing annoyed, cautious, and fumbling in his nonverbal behavior (in all cases, the actor appeared on camera with a script in hand). Pretesting showed that the differences conveyed were substantial. Half the participants in each demeanor condition were pre-instructed that they would see the actual witness testify: "What you see now is Dennis Ottway testifying in court at the actual trial." Assigned to the reader condition, the other half were told that the actual witness could not attend and that "the person you will see answering the questions is not Dennis Ottway but a clerk who was designated to read Mr. Ottway's statement." In a fifth control group, participants merely read the transcript.

The results were unambiguous. Manipulation checks showed that participants were fully aware of whether they were watching the witness himself or a surrogate reader. Yet strong main effects for demeanor, unqualified by any two-way interactions, revealed that jurors in the positive versus negative demeanor condition perceived the witness's testimony as more accurate and credible, and altered their verdicts accordingly—even in the reader condition! It is this latter finding that I termed the "messenger effect" in persuasion (indicating the limits of this effect, the reader's demeanor did not similarly corrupt the perceived *character* of the actual witness).

Conceptually, this effect feels like a close cousin to the fundamental attribution error by which social perceivers take behavior at face value without sufficient appreciation of contextual factors. That people cannot evaluate the content of a source's message independent of the speaker who delivers it had obvious implications for courtroom procedure and the use of videotaped depositions. But I have always thought that this distinction touched on an important—and yes, underappreciated—aspect of persuasion. Many communicators both in life and in the laboratory are the origin or source of the message they deliver, as in the preacher, the expert witness, the editorial writer, and the doctor who recommends a new way to brush your teeth. Other communicators are mere messengers, however, relatively unattached to the source, as in the surrogate witness or the celebrity hired to advertise a commercial product. But what about the press secretary, the U.N. ambassador, the attorney who represents a client in court, or the company spokesperson who delivers a message that is approved by the source he or she represents? To what extent is the source in these cases boosted or undermined by the messenger's demeanor? I had envisioned a number of follow-up studies to address an array of interesting empirical questions (e.g., varying the relationship between a messenger and source, the physical appearance of the messenger as well as demeanor). But then I became entranced by the social psychology of false confessions, which, interestingly, present a source misattribution dilemma of a different sort, as judges and juries seek to determine how an apparently innocent person could have self-incriminated and exhibited guilty knowledge in his or her narrative statement.

Well, no one else came forward to pick up on my hidden gem. Note that "hidden" is the operative word: To date, this article has been cited a grand total of three times—now four.

REFERENCES

Kassin, S. M. (1983). Deposition testimony and the surrogate witness: Evidence for a "messenger effect" in persuasion. *Personality and Social Psychology Bulletin, 9*, 281–288.
Kassin, S. M. (1984). Mock jury trials. *Trial Diplomacy Journal, 7*, 26–30.
Kassin, S. M., & Wrightsman, L. S. (1988). *The American jury on trial: Psychological perspectives.* Washington, DC: Hemisphere.

JAMES W. PENNEBAKER, University of Texas at Austin

The Idea, The Audience, and Me

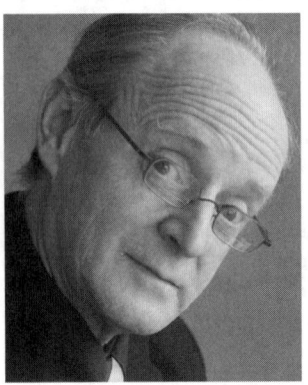

As with everyone in this book, I have had many good—OK, brilliant, really—
ideas slammed by grant and journal reviewers, editors, friends, and even
family members. I've published articles that I thought were stunning that had no
impact. And I've given an occasional talk that I was convinced was potentially
groundbreaking, only to receive polite applause. It can be a brutal world, but, ultimately, the free market of ideas must be respected.

If the idea didn't connect with the audience, it was probably the fault of the idea,
or the audience, but in either case, it was my own failure to mold the idea into a
story that was appropriate to that particular audience. So, from this vantage point, I
haven't had many truly underappreciated ideas. Rather, I've been the author of
some things that were either weak (and therefore were not appreciated appropriately) or that I didn't package well enough for the audience I was addressing.

FAILED IDEAS: EXAMPLES AND INTERPRETATIONS

Most of my ideas that were initially underappreciated were eventually published.
Sometimes, the editors or reviewers erred (you know who you are); other times,

the mistake was mine alone, and I then revised the manuscript to tell a better story. There were a few studies, however, that just didn't sell. Indeed, some never even made it to manuscript status. Here are a few.

Classical Conditioning of Begonias

As a graduate student, I borrowed a fellow student's begonia plant to see if it was possible to apply principles of temporal conditioning on the leaves of the plant. Measuring the action potential of the leaves with a sophisticated polygraph machine, I found evidence that the begonia reacted to light fluctuations in a manner consistent with classical conditioning. I was ridiculed by so many fellow graduate students that it became clear that my career might be in jeopardy if I continued this work. The owner of the begonia plant, one Charles Carver, was so furious about my treatment of his plant that it took years for us to reconcile our friendship.

Hindsight analysis: Ideas that challenge basic views about the world are rarely well received. To have continued this line of work would have required a level of persistence that didn't make sense at the time. Pursuing interesting but possibly crackpot ideas prior to tenure is a very bad idea.

Control Over Your Own Body

My still-unpublished doctoral dissertation found that people's beliefs about their control over bodily functions could influence their actual control. If a person was made to feel that he or she had control over a biological process, instructions to exert control made it very difficult to do. If people were led to believe that they had no control over a biological function, instructions to influence that function were more successful.

Hindsight analysis: The idea was too complex and relied on an out-of-favor theoretical framework. The average reviewer simply could not relate to the theory or phenomenon.

Men and Women Talk Differently

This one seemed like a no-brainer. Averaging across thousands of text files representing multiple genres (e.g., natural conversation, expressive writing, composition of poems or novels), women and men use words differently. Even when writing about the same topics, women use first-person-singular pronouns and cognitive words more than do men. Men use articles and prepositions more. These are not subtle effects, and, in dozens of surveys of very smart people, very few people predict these findings. The paper (Newman et al., 2008) was rejected by every major journal in psychology and social psychology—for years. No two rejections were the same. It was finally published in *Discourse Processes* and is the most downloaded paper I have published in the past decade.

Hindsight analysis: Like the mental life of begonias, statements about sex differences uncover political, philosophical, and deep-seated emotional issues in audiences that can be hard to bridge. I'm also culpable in that I did not have a strong theoretical or political stake in the effects. Had I framed the paper as evidence for or against an evolutionary or social constructivist position, I may have marshaled enough support from committed reviewers to get the paper accepted in a top-tier journal.

ON MAKING AN APPRECIATED IDEA

What makes for an idea that is appreciated by others? It has to be a good idea, generally speaking, and it must be framed well. And did I mention that it helps if the idea is in a paper that is well written and enjoyable to read? In my experience, a truly appreciated idea—one that resonates with people—is one that is simple, directly relevant to the real world as people experience it, and, ideally, makes people see that world differently, in new ways.

Simplicity

Think of the greatest studies in psychology. The ones that influenced me the most were Milgram's obedience studies, Asch's social influence projects, Darley and Latané's bystander studies, and Schachter and Singer's two-factor theory of emotion. These were not complex experiments that relied on esoteric statistics. They all made simple and straightforward points that could be reduced to a sentence or two.

Not only were the designs simple, but so were the statistics. A great idea is one that can be conveyed in a single sentence, perhaps two. If the underlying statistics require mediational or moderating variables, complex modeling, or other esoteric statistics, it is unlikely that the underlying idea will have much staying power. It may well be accepted in a top journal, but very few people will understand it or care about it. A good idea is one that is simple and straightforward.

Real-World Relevance

I was drawn to psychology because it is a theoretical discipline that could, in principle, have an impact on people in my lifetime. For an idea to have punch, other people—both within and outside psychology—should be able to appreciate it when they hear about it. Whether scientists or laypeople, most audiences sense when an idea is tethered to something tangible, and useful, in everyday life.

Perhaps the best test of the relevance of an idea is to talk with someone who is not steeped in your own research tradition. As you explain your theory or results, do your friends' eyes glaze over? Bad sign. If, however, they perk up and start asking questions, your idea might be as good as you thought. As a side note, people's questions about research can be invaluable. The questions that people ask can inform you about what your next logical research question might be.

Challenging the Conventional Wisdom

There is a difference between an appreciated idea and a published one. The goal, of course, is to meld them into one. The reality is that some of the field's most appreciated studies have been controversial. Powerful ideas often threaten the status quo. Consider some of the most influential and controversial ideas in social psychology—terror management theory, evolutionary psychology, and the work on implicit attitudes. Love them or not, these perspectives get under the skin of some of our colleagues. We don't have to like or accept the theories, but the approaches are broadly appreciated. They get all of us to stop and pay attention.

Persistence

It is safe to say that the 50 authors of this volume have had more papers rejected and grants turned down than the average social psychologist. Those who have published the most appreciated ideas probably also have been told, on many occasions, that their ideas came up short or their data were only half-baked. To the degree that your idea is simple and relevant and challenges the conventional wisdom, there is a very good chance that it will face an uphill battle in the early stages of the publication game. I would wager that those ideas most appreciated in the field today were among those that started off as among the least appreciated.

REFERENCE

Newman, M. L., Groom, C. J., Handelman, L. D., & Pennebaker, J. W. (2008). Gender differences in language use: An analysis of 14,000 text samples. *Discourse Processes, 45,* 211–4246.

JERALD JELLISON, University of Southern California, retired

Unfinished Business: Activating Change

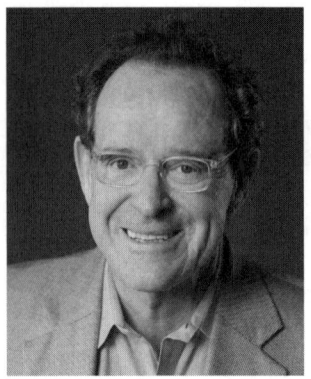

On a whim 30 years ago, I volunteered to join the Board of Directors of the USC Credit Union. Credit unions are cooperatives and are comparable to banks. Fate moved again in two years, when I was pressured to become President of the USC Credit Union. With insufficient wisdom and unwarranted confidence, I took my first steps into the business world.

We were a small, barely profitable organization with only $2 million in assets. Growth was imperative. We needed to expand our limited hours of operation (10 to 12 and 1 to 3). The lunch hour, when all of our 2.5 employees were eating in the student union, was exactly the time faculty and staff members wanted to handle financial matters. To open between 12 and 1, Ethel, our bookkeeper, would have to learn the duties of a part-time teller.

One day I invited Ethel to the student union for a cup of coffee. My goal was to persuade her to do the cross-training necessary for the new responsibilities. I established my credibility, explained the logic of the extended hours, and finished with what I thought was an emotionally compelling picture of how she could help the organization grow by learning to serve as a fill-in teller. After our third visit to the student union, I realized no matter how much I talked, or how many coffees I plied her with, Ethel's answer would remain a firm "no." This was devastating. The best social psychological principles of influence had failed.

As my business experience increased, I saw many examples of the limitations of changing people's behavior by first trying to change their attitudes. What was the problem? In simple terms, people's resistance to change has emotional roots, and changing their cognitions is ineffective against these affective barriers. It's similar to an idea proposed years ago by Sherif and Hovland (1954). On any attitude issue, individuals have a range of positions they're willing to accept and a range of positions they reject. These theorists asserted that while persuasion can change attitudes inside a person's range or latitude of attitudinal acceptance, it is ineffective in getting people to accept a position located in their latitude of rejection. Negative emotions divide the acceptable and the unacceptable attitude positions.

To understand the emotional dynamics of behavior change, try charting the psychological trajectory of change along a J curve. You can represent it graphically by drawing the letter "J." Next, add a flat line, straight out to the left from the top of the short arm of the J to connect with the Y axis of a graph. This flat portion is the starting point. Performance is stable because the person is successfully doing things in a well-established pattern. Using a topographic metaphor, change requires leaving the flat plateau, dropping down into the valley of the J, and then climbing the long arm of the J to the top of the mountain.

Moving from the safety of the plateau involves going over a precipice. This is the most difficult part of the change process because it's extremely frightening to go over the emotional cliff. For resisters, change doesn't mean jumping into the unknown—they can easily imagine the horrors at the bottom of the sheer drop.

These fears can be overcome with a behavior-oriented influence strategy called activation (Jellison, 2006). While Festinger's (1954) theory of dissonance described one-way behavior change can cause attitude change, activation provides a systematic and practical approach. It consists of techniques that help people start taking action despite their doubts and fears. Once people take the initial steps, they usually discover two things. First, their worst fears aren't realistic (e.g., think how we turn on a light to calm a frightened child and prove there aren't any monsters in the room), and second, they begin to experience some success doing things the new way. When people personally experience the benefits of change, they develop positive attitudes and feelings.

Persuasive communications describe the benefits of changing, while activation lets people actually savor these rewards. The logic of persuasion is to change attitudes in order to influence behavior. Activation reverses the process by instigating small behavior changes, which lead to larger changes in behavior as well as positive feelings and attitudes.

Without understanding the social psychological dynamics, businesspeople have been using activation for years. It's called the free sample. Imagine receiving a small container of a new shampoo. Although you're satisfied with your current brand, you take the free sample along for your weekend at the cabin. In the shower Saturday morning, you open the container and inhale an intoxicating aroma. Even a small amount produces abundant lather, and afterward your hair is tangle-free and easy to shape. After these positive experiences, you stop at a drugstore on the way home and purchase a bottle.

Automobile salespeople often use activation. You want an efficient car for commuting, but you end up buying a more expensive model. Why? Most likely it was the test drive. Driving the car and experiencing its responsiveness, plus touching and smelling the leather interior, all while listening to the sound system produced the change.

The first key element in activation is making the initial actions simple and easy. These so-called baby steps must be described in very specific language—ground-level words. With Ethel at the credit union, we stopped using high-altitude phrases such as "expand your skill set," "learn to multitask," and "become a team player." Instead we asked her to spend three minutes watching Betina, the main teller, simply log on and off the computer. Ethel's only action was to watch. The next day, Betina assisted Ethel as she logged on and off for five minutes. Many more small steps followed.

Small obstacles can cause resisters to raise their defenses. Therefore, even the slightest of barriers should be removed. Each session was so brief it didn't interfere with Ethel's primary duties and didn't cause her to stay longer at the end of the day.

The possibility of failure can arouse fears about trying something new. The fear of looking foolish or suffering even worse consequences can cause people to stick with something they know will produce marginally successful results. With a metaphoric safety net, people are much more willing to take a risk. Reassure the person that mistakes are to be expected and are acceptable at the beginning because they accelerate the learning process. Betina never criticized Ethel's actions. Instead, she used encouraging phrases such as "very good, for your first try"; "that's much better, now let's try to improve even more"; "that's fine, but this time enter the deposit code before the transaction amount."

Activation also incorporates the social psychological principle of getting people involved in making decisions about the process of change. The leader may decide which mountain to climb, and even which face of the mountain to ascend, but the hikers can participate in making small decisions that arise on the trail. In each training session, Ethel was asked which of the different skill sets she wanted to learn next.

If you reflect on the J curve, when does it really become profitable to make a change? It's toward the end, when the new performance level exceeds the original plateau. Although the nature of life dictates that the big benefits of change come at the end, human nature demands the rewards right now. Because people initially make many errors and frequently stumble down the side of the cliff, they don't receive many benefits. This is the time to "front-load rewards."

At the beginning, Ethel's efforts alone garnered praise, regardless of whether she was successful. Fractional components of her actions were lauded, "That was great. You remembered the code number." When she successfully completed the initial stage of training, she earned a gift certificate.

The move from practice sessions to actually serving customers instigated a new J curve, and the entire activation process was repeated. With Betina by her side, Ethel worked the teller line for 15 minutes, then 30, then 60. Ethel soon felt confident and competent. After a week of noon-time teller duty, Ethel discovered she liked the time outside her cubicle, and she enjoyed talking directly with people. She soon developed friendships with several regular customers. While the change was instigated to help the organization, Ethel discovered it also worked to her personal benefit.

Praise and other external incentives are initially used to induce behavior change, but with success, people will discover unexpected ways the new behavior pattern aligns with their own self-interest (e.g., Ethel made new friends). External incentives may instigate the new behavior, but soon it will become intrinsically appealing.

Each element of activation is directed at minimizing fear and any other negative emotions that produce resistance. Small do-able steps are much less frightening than thinking about climbing to the mountaintop. Knowing it's okay to make mistakes minimizes another major source of fear. By involving people in implementation of the change, they gain a sense of control, which also reduces their fear. Removing barriers and front-loading rewards helps neutralize the negative feelings that can impede change.

In the beginning, activation was designed as an influence technique to help managers encourage resistant employees to adopt innovative business practices (it's also useful in getting bosses to change). Since then it has been applied in many situations: promoting health practices, facilitating people's adaptation to new jobs and new bosses, improving customer service, and even religious conversion.

Although activation is grounded in social psychological principles, it hasn't been systematically studied. It's underappreciated because the idea was originally published in a business book and therefore is unknown to academic psychologists. I urge active researchers to examine the underlying dynamics and parameters of this practical approach to influence.

Activation has implications for many theoretical topics. It provides a unique perspective on the link between attitudes and behavior, as discussed in this volume by Icek Ajzen in Chapter 3. While social psychology has explored the superiority of intrinsic motivation over extrinsic motivation, the activation concept addresses the issue of how people originally become intrinsically motivated to perform certain actions. Activation implies that extrinsic incentives can play a critical role in establishing new behavior patterns that then become intrinsically satisfying.

From the early days of getting Ethel to change, the USC Credit Union has grown to over $400 million in assets, and I continue to volunteer my services as Chairman of the Board. Over the years, I also became involved in other business ventures and retired early from USC to concentrate on helping managers learn the activation approach to implementing change. I found this second career so challenging and satisfying that I wrote a book (Jellison, 2010) to help graduate students, and professors, make the transition from academics to business. Whether you're switching careers, or confronting resistance, activation is a practical way to make change happen.

REFERENCES

Festinger, L. (1957). *A theory of cognitive dissonance.* Palo Alto, CA: Stanford University Press.

Jellison, J. (2006). *Managing the dynamics of change.* New York: McGraw Hill.

Jellison, J. (2010). *Life after grad school.* New York: Oxford University Press.

Sherif, M., & Hovland, C. (1961). *Social judgment: Assimilation and contrast effects in communication and attitude change.* New Haven: Yale University Press.